3 HESI Admission Assessment Practice Tests

Three Practice Tests for the HESI Admission Assessment (A2) Exam

TABLE OF CONTENTS

Exam Overview

Every nursing program is different, and you may or may not be tested on all of the following sections:

- <u>Math:</u> 50-item exam. Focuses on math needed for calculation of Drugs and Solutions. 50 minutes.
- <u>Reading Comprehension</u>: 47-item exam. Reading scenarios that are health related. The reading scenarios pop up on the screen. Students can move around the windows to see the entire scenario. 50 minutes
- <u>Vocabulary and General Knowledge</u>: 50-item exam. Contains basic vocabulary that is often used in health care fields. 50 minutes.
- <u>Grammar</u>: 50-item exam. Contains basic grammar. Time allotment: 50 minutes
- <u>Chemistry</u>: 25-item exam. 25 minutes.
- <u>Anatomy and Physiology (A&P)</u>: 25-item exam. 25 minutes.
- <u>Biology</u>: 25-item exam. 25 minutes.
- Not Scored Sections:
- <u>Learning Styles</u>: Identifies individual learning style and prints test-taking and study tips best suited for the individual's learning style and relates these recommendations to nursing curricula.
- <u>Personality Style:</u> Uses concepts related to introversion and extroversion to classify the student's personality style. Explanations are printed at the conclusion of the exam to let the student know how to use his/her personality style to be successful in a nursing education program.

HESI A²PracticeTest#1

Reading Comprehension	Vocabulary and General Knowledge	Grammar	Mathematics
1. _____	1. _____ 49. _____	1. _____ 49. _____	1. _____ 49. _____
2. _____	2. _____ 50. _____	2. _____ 50. _____	2. _____ 50. _____
3. _____	3. _____	3. _____	3. _____
4. _____	4. _____	4. _____	4. _____
5. _____	5. _____	5. _____	5. _____
6. _____	6. _____	6. _____	6. _____
7. _____	7. _____	7. _____	7. _____
8. _____	8. _____	8. _____	8. _____
9. _____	9. _____	9. _____	9. _____
10. _____	10. _____	10. _____	10. _____
11. _____	11. _____	11. _____	11. _____
12. _____	12. _____	12. _____	12. _____
13. _____	13. _____	13. _____	13. _____
14. _____	14. _____	14. _____	14. _____
15. _____	15. _____	15. _____	15. _____
16. _____	16. _____	16. _____	16. _____
17. _____	17. _____	17. _____	17. _____
18. _____	18. _____	18. _____	18. _____
19. _____	19. _____	19. _____	19. _____
20. _____	20. _____	20. _____	20. _____
21. _____	21. _____	21. _____	21. _____
22. _____	22. _____	22. _____	22. _____
23. _____	23. _____	23. _____	23. _____
24. _____	24. _____	24. _____	24. _____
25. _____	25. _____	25. _____	25. _____
26. _____	26. _____	26. _____	26. _____
27. _____	27. _____	27. _____	27. _____
28. _____	28. _____	28. _____	28. _____
29. _____	29. _____	29. _____	29. _____
30. _____	30. _____	30. _____	30. _____
31. _____	31. _____	31. _____	31. _____
32. _____	32. _____	32. _____	32. _____
33. _____	33. _____	33. _____	33. _____
34. _____	34. _____	34. _____	34. _____
35. _____	35. _____	35. _____	35. _____
36. _____	36. _____	36. _____	36. _____
37. _____	37. _____	37. _____	37. _____
38. _____	38. _____	38. _____	38. _____
39. _____	39. _____	39. _____	39. _____
40. _____	40. _____	40. _____	40. _____
41. _____	41. _____	41. _____	41. _____
42. _____	42. _____	42. _____	42. _____
43. _____	43. _____	43. _____	43. _____
44. _____	44. _____	44. _____	44. _____
45. _____	45. _____	45. _____	45. _____
46. _____	46. _____	46. _____	46. _____
47. _____	47. _____	47. _____	47. _____
	48. _____	48. _____	48. _____

Biology	Chemistry	Anatomy and Physiology
1. _____	1. _____	1. _____
2. _____	2. _____	2. _____
3. _____	3. _____	3. _____
4. _____	4. _____	4. _____
5. _____	5. _____	5. _____
6. _____	6. _____	6. _____
7. _____	7. _____	7. _____
8. _____	8. _____	8. _____
9. _____	9. _____	9. _____
10. _____	10. _____	10. _____
11. _____	11. _____	11. _____
12. _____	12. _____	12. _____
13. _____	13. _____	13. _____
14. _____	14. _____	14. _____
15. _____	15. _____	15. _____
16. _____	16. _____	16. _____
17. _____	17. _____	17. _____
18. _____	18. _____	18. _____
19. _____	19. _____	19. _____
20. _____	20. _____	20. _____
21. _____	21. _____	21. _____
22. _____	22. _____	22. _____
23. _____	23. _____	23. _____
24. _____	24. _____	24. _____
25. _____	25. _____	25. _____

<table>
<tr><td><h1>Section 1. Reading Comprehension</h1></td><td>Number of Questions: **47**

Time Limit: **50 Minutes**</td></tr>
</table>

Questions 1 to 4 pertain to the following passage:

It is most likely that you have never had diphtheria. You probably don't even know anyone who has suffered from this disease. In fact, you may not even know what diphtheria is. Similarly, diseases like whooping cough, measles, mumps, and rubella may all be unfamiliar to you. In the nineteenth and early twentieth centuries, these illnesses struck hundreds of thousands of people in the United States each year, mostly children, and tens of thousands of people died. The names of these diseases were frightening household words. Today, they are all but forgotten. That change happened largely because of vaccines.

You probably have been vaccinated against diphtheria. You may even have been exposed to the bacterium that causes it, but the vaccine prepared your body to fight off the disease so quickly that you were unaware of the infection. Vaccines take advantage of your body's natural ability to learn how to combat many disease-causing germs, or microbes. What's more, your body remembers how to protect itself from the microbes it has encountered before. Collectively, the parts of your body that remember and repel microbes are called the immune system. Without the proper functioning of the immune system, the simplest illness—even the common cold—could quickly turn deadly.

On average, your immune system needs more than a week to learn how to fight off an unfamiliar microbe. Sometimes, that isn't enough time. Strong microbes can spread through your body faster than the immune system can fend them off. Your body often gains the upper hand after a few weeks, but in the meantime you are sick. Certain microbes are so virulent that they can overwhelm or escape your natural defenses. In those situations, vaccines can make all the difference.

Traditional vaccines contain either parts of microbes or whole microbes that have been altered so that they don't cause disease. When your immune system confronts these harmless versions of the germs, it quickly clears them from your body. In other words, vaccines trick your immune system in order to teach your body important lessons about how to defeat its opponents.

1. What is the main idea of the passage?
   A. The nineteenth and early twentieth centuries were a dark period for medicine.
   B. You have probably never had diphtheria.
   C. Traditional vaccines contain altered microbes.
   D. Vaccines help the immune system function properly.

2. Which statement is *not* a detail from the passage?
   A. Vaccines contain microbe parts or altered microbes.
   B. The immune system typically needs a week to learn how to fight a new disease.
   C. The symptoms of disease do not emerge until the body has learned how to fight the microbe.
   D. A hundred years ago, children were at the greatest risk of dying from now-treatable diseases.

3. What is the meaning of the word *virulent* as it is used in the third paragraph?
   A. tiny
   B. malicious
   C. contagious
   D. annoying

4. What is the author's primary purpose in writing the essay?
   A. to entertain
   B. to persuade
   C. to inform
   D. to analyze

Questions 5 to 8 pertain to the following passage:

Foodborne illnesses are contracted by eating food or drinking beverages contaminated with bacteria, parasites, or viruses. Harmful chemicals can also cause foodborne illnesses if they have contaminated food during harvesting or processing. Foodborne illnesses can cause symptoms ranging from upset stomach to diarrhea, fever, vomiting, abdominal cramps, and dehydration. Most foodborne infections are undiagnosed and unreported, though the Centers for Disease Control and Prevention estimates that every year about 76 million people in the United States become ill from pathogens in food. About 5,000 of these people die.

Harmful bacteria are the most common cause of foodborne illness. Some bacteria may be present at the point of purchase. Raw foods are the most common source of foodborne illnesses because they are not sterile; examples include raw meat and poultry contaminated during slaughter. Seafood may become contaminated during harvest or processing. One in 10,000 eggs may be contaminated with Salmonella inside the shell. Produce, such as spinach, lettuce, tomatoes, sprouts, and melons, can become contaminated with Salmonella, Shigella, or Escherichia coli (E. coli). Contamination can occur during growing, harvesting, processing, storing, shipping, or final preparation. Sources of produce contamination vary, as these foods are grown in soil and can become contaminated during growth, processing, or distribution. Contamination may also occur during food preparation in a restaurant or a home kitchen. The most common form of contamination from handled foods is the calicivirus, also called the Norwalk-like virus.

When food is cooked and left out for more than two hours at room temperature, bacteria can multiply quickly. Most bacteria don't produce an odor or change in color or texture, so they can be impossible to detect. Freezing food slows or stops bacteria's growth, but does not destroy the bacteria. The microbes can become reactivated when the food is thawed. Refrigeration also can slow the growth of some bacteria. Thorough cooking is required to destroy the bacteria.

5. What is the subject of the passage?
   A. foodborne illnesses
   B. the dangers of uncooked food
   C. bacteria
   D. proper food preparation

6. Which statement is *not* a detail from the passage?
   A. Every year, more than 70 million Americans contract some form of foodborne illness.
   B. Once food is cooked, it cannot cause illness.
   C. Refrigeration can slow the growth of some bacteria.
   D. The most common form of contamination in handled foods is calicivirus.

7. What is the meaning of the word *pathogens* as it is used in the first paragraph?
   A. diseases
   B. vaccines
   C. disease-causing substances
   D. foods

8. What is the meaning of the word *sterile* as it is used in the second paragraph?
   A. free of bacteria
   B. healthy
   C. delicious
   D. impotent

Questions 9 to 12 pertain to the following passage:

There are a number of health problems related to bleeding in the esophagus and stomach. Stomach acid can cause inflammation and bleeding at the lower end of the esophagus. This condition, usually associated with the symptom of heartburn, is called esophagitis, or inflammation of the esophagus. Sometimes a muscle between the esophagus and stomach fails to close properly and allows the return of food and stomach juices into the esophagus, which can lead to esophagitis. In another unrelated condition, enlarged veins (varices) at the lower end of the esophagus rupture and bleed massively. Cirrhosis of the liver is the most common cause of esophageal varices. Esophageal bleeding can be caused by a tear in the lining of the esophagus (Mallory-Weiss syndrome). Mallory-Weiss syndrome usually results from vomiting, but may also be caused by increased pressure in the abdomen from coughing, hiatal hernia, or childbirth. Esophageal cancer can cause bleeding.

The stomach is a frequent site of bleeding. Infections with Helicobacter pylori (H. pylori), alcohol, aspirin, aspirin-containing medicines, and various other medicines (such as nonsteroidal anti-inflammatory drugs [NSAIDs]—particularly those used for arthritis) can cause stomach ulcers or inflammation (gastritis). The stomach is often the site of ulcer disease. Acute or chronic ulcers may enlarge and erode through a blood vessel, causing bleeding. Also, patients suffering from burns, shock, head injuries, cancer, or those who have undergone extensive surgery may develop stress ulcers. Bleeding can also occur from benign tumors or cancer of the stomach, although these disorders usually do not cause massive bleeding.

9. What is the main idea of the passage?
   A. The digestive system is complex.
   B. Of all the digestive organs, the stomach is the most prone to bleeding.
   C. Both the esophagus and the stomach are subject to bleeding problems.
   D. Esophagitis afflicts the young and old alike.

10. Which statement is *not* a detail from the passage?
   A. Alcohol can cause stomach bleeding.
   B. Ulcer disease rarely occurs in the stomach.
   C. Benign tumors rarely result in massive bleeding.
   D. Childbirth is one cause of Mallory-Weiss syndrome.

11. What is the meaning of the word *rupture* as it is used in the first paragraph?
   A. tear
   B. collapse
   C. implode
   D. detach

12. What is the meaning of the word *erode* as it is used in the second paragraph?
   A. avoid
   B. divorce
   C. contain
   D. wear away

Questions 13 to 16 pertain to the following passage:

We met Kathy Blake while she was taking a stroll in the park . . . by herself. What's so striking about this is that Kathy is completely blind, and she has been for more than 30 years.

The diagnosis from her doctor was retinitis pigmentosa, or RP. It's an incurable genetic disease that leads to progressive visual loss. Photoreceptive cells in the retina slowly start to die, leaving the patient visually impaired.

"Life was great the year before I was diagnosed," Kathy said. "I had just started a new job; I just bought my first new car. I had just started dating my now-husband. Life was good. The doctor had told me that there was some good news and some bad news. 'The bad news is you are going to lose your vision; the good news is we don't think you are going to go totally blind.' Unfortunately, I did lose all my vision within about 15 years."

Two years ago, Kathy got a glimmer of hope. She heard about an artificial retina being developed in Los Angeles. It was experimental, but Kathy was the perfect candidate.

Dr. Mark Humayun is a retinal surgeon and biomedical engineer. "A good candidate for the artificial retina device is a person who is blind because of retinal blindness," he said. "They've lost the rods and cones, the light-sensing cells of the eye, but the rest of the circuitry is relatively intact. In the simplest rendition, this device basically takes a blind person and hooks them up to a camera."

It may sound like the stuff of science fiction . . . and just a few years ago it was. A camera is built into a pair of glasses, sending radio signals to a tiny chip in the back of the retina. The chip, small enough to fit on a fingertip, is implanted surgically and stimulates the nerves that lead to the vision center of the brain. Kathy is one of twenty patients who have undergone surgery and use the device.

It has been about two years since the surgery, and Kathy still comes in for weekly testing at the University of Southern California's medical campus. She scans back and forth with specially made, camera-equipped glasses until she senses objects on a screen and then touches the objects. The low-resolution image from the camera is still enough to make out the black stripes on the screen. Impulses are sent from the camera to the 60 receptors that are on the chip in her retina. So, what is Kathy seeing?

"I see flashes of light that indicate a contrast from light to dark—very similar to a camera flash, probably not quite as bright because it's not hurting my eye at all," she replied.

Humayun underscored what a breakthrough this is and how a patient adjusts. "If you've been blind for 30 or 50 years, (and) all of a sudden you get this device, there is a period of learning," he said. "Your brain needs to learn. And it's literally like seeing a baby crawl—to a child walk—to an adult run."

While hardly perfect, the device works best in bright light or where there is a lot of contrast. Kathy takes the device home. The software that runs the device can be upgraded. So, as the software is upgraded, her vision improves. Recently, she was outside with her husband on a moonlit night and saw something she hadn't seen for a long time.

"I scanned up in the sky (and) I got a big flash, right where the moon was, and pointed it out. I can't even remember how many years ago it's been that I would have ever been able to do that."

This technology has a bright future. The current chip has a resolution of 60 pixels. Humayun says that number could be increased to more than a thousand in the next version.

"I think it will be extremely exciting if they can recognize their loved ones' faces and be able to see what their wife or husband or their grandchildren look like, which they haven't seen," said Humayun.

Kathy dreams of a day when blindness like hers will be a distant memory. "My eye disease is hereditary," she said. "My three daughters happen to be fine, but I want to know that if my grandchildren ever have a problem, they will have something to give them some vision."

13. What is the primary subject of the passage?
    A. a new artificial retina
    B. Kathy Blake
    C. hereditary disease
    D. Dr. Mark Humayun

14. What is the meaning of the word *progressive* as it is used in the second paragraph?
    A. selective
    B. gradually increasing
    C. diminishing
    D. disabling

15. Which statement is *not* a detail from the passage?
    A. The use of an artificial retina requires a special pair of glasses.
    B. Retinal blindness is the inability to perceive light.
    C. Retinitis pigmentosa is curable.
    D. The artificial retina performs best in bright light.

16. What is the author's intention in writing the essay?
    A. to persuade
    B. to entertain
    C. to analyze
    D. to inform

Questions 17 to 21 pertain to the following passage:

Usher syndrome is the most common condition that affects both hearing and vision. The major symptoms of Usher syndrome are hearing loss and an eye disorder called retinitis pigmentosa, or RP. Retinitis pigmentosa causes night blindness and a loss of peripheral vision (side vision) through the progressive degeneration of the retina. The retina, which is crucial for vision, is a light-sensitive tissue at the back of the eye. As RP progresses, the field of vision narrows, until only central vision (the ability to see straight ahead) remains. Many people with Usher syndrome also have severe balance problems.

There are three clinical types of Usher syndrome. In the United States, types 1 and 2 are the most common. Together, they account for approximately 90 to 95 percent of all cases of juvenile Usher syndrome. Approximately three to six percent of all deaf and hearing-disabled children have Usher syndrome. In developed countries, such as the United States, about four in every 100,000 newborns have Usher syndrome.

Usher syndrome is inherited as an autosomal recessive trait. The term autosomal means that the mutated gene is not located on either of the chromosomes that determine sex; in other words, both males and females can have the disorder and can pass it along to a child. The word recessive means that in order to have Usher syndrome, an individual must receive a mutated form of the Usher syndrome gene from each parent. If a child has a mutation in one Usher syndrome gene but the other gene is normal, he or she should have normal vision and hearing. Individuals with a mutation in a gene that can cause an autosomal recessive disorder are called carriers, because they carry the mutated gene but show no symptoms of the disorder. If both parents are carriers of a mutated gene for Usher syndrome, they will have a one-in-four chance of producing a child with Usher syndrome.

Usually, parents who have normal hearing and vision do not know if they are carriers of an Usher syndrome gene mutation. Currently, it is not possible to determine whether an individual without a family history of Usher syndrome is a carrier. Scientists at the National Institute on Deafness and Other Communication Disorders (NIDCD) are hoping to change this, however, as they learn more about the genes responsible for Usher syndrome.

17. What is the main idea of the passage?
    A. Usher syndrome is an inherited condition that affects hearing and vision.
    B. Some people are carriers of Usher syndrome.
    C. Usher syndrome typically skips a generation.
    D. Scientists hope to develop a test for detecting the carriers of Usher syndrome.

18. What is the meaning of the word *symptoms* as it is used in the first paragraph?
    A. qualifications
    B. conditions
    C. disorders
    D. perceptible signs

19. Which statement is *not* a detail from the passage?
    A. Types 1 and 2 Usher syndrome are the most common in the United States.
    B. Usher syndrome affects both hearing and smell.
    C. Right now, there is no way to identify a carrier of Usher syndrome.
    D. Central vision is the ability to see straight ahead.

20. What is the meaning of the word *juvenile* as it is used in the second paragraph?
    A. bratty
    B. serious
    C. occurring in children
    D. improper

21. What is the meaning of the word *mutated* as it is used in the third paragraph?
    A. selected
    B. altered
    C. composed
    D. destroyed

Questions 22 to 27 pertain to the following passage:
   The immune system is a network of cells, tissues, and organs that defends the body against attacks by foreign invaders. These invaders are primarily microbes—tiny organisms such as bacteria, parasites, and fungi—that can cause infections. Viruses also cause infections, but are too primitive to be classified as living organisms. The human body provides an ideal environment for many microbes. It is the immune system's job to keep the microbes out or destroy them.
   The immune system is amazingly complex. It can recognize and remember millions of different enemies, and it can secrete fluids and cells to wipe out nearly all of them. The secret to its success is an elaborate and dynamic communications network. Millions of cells, organized into sets and subsets, gather and transfer information in response to an infection. Once immune cells receive the alarm, they produce powerful chemicals that help to regulate their own growth and behavior, enlist other immune cells, and direct the new recruits to trouble spots.
   Although scientists have learned much about the immune system, they continue to puzzle over how the body destroys invading microbes, infected cells, and tumors without harming healthy tissues. New technologies for identifying individual immune cells are now allowing scientists to determine quickly which targets are triggering an immune response. Improvements in microscopy are permitting the first-ever observations of living B cells, T cells, and other cells as they interact within lymph nodes and other body tissues.
   In addition, scientists are rapidly unraveling the genetic blueprints that direct the human immune response, as well as those that dictate the biology of bacteria, viruses, and

parasites. The combination of new technology with expanded genetic information will no doubt reveal even more about how the body protects itself from disease.

22. What is the main idea of the passage?
    A. Scientists fully understand the immune system.
    B. The immune system triggers the production of fluids.
    C. The body is under constant invasion by malicious microbes.
    D. The immune system protects the body from infection.

23. Which statement is *not* a detail from the passage?
    A. Most invaders of the body are microbes.
    B. The immune system relies on excellent communication.
    C. Viruses are extremely sophisticated.
    D. The cells of the immune system are organized.

24. What is the meaning of the word *ideal* as it is used in the first paragraph?
    A. thoughtful
    B. confined
    C. hostile
    D. perfect

25. Which statement is *not* a detail from the passage?
    A. Scientists can now see T cells.
    B. The immune system ignores tumors.
    C. The ability of the immune system to fight disease without harming the body remains mysterious.
    D. The immune system remembers millions of different invaders.

26. What is the meaning of the word *enlist* as it is used in the second paragraph?
    A. call into service
    B. write down
    C. send away
    D. put across

27. What is the author's primary purpose in writing the essay?
    A. to persuade
    B. to analyze
    C. to inform
    D. to entertain

Questions 28 to 31 pertain to the following passage:
    The federal government regulates dietary supplements through the United States Food and Drug Administration (FDA). The regulations for dietary supplements are not the same as those for prescription or over-the-counter drugs. In general, the regulations for dietary supplements are less strict.
    To begin with, a manufacturer does not have to prove the safety and effectiveness of a dietary supplement before it is marketed. A manufacturer is permitted to say that a dietary supplement addresses a nutrient deficiency, supports health, or is linked to a particular body function (such as immunity), if there is research to support the claim. Such a claim must be followed by the words "This statement has not been evaluated by the Food and Drug Administration. This product is not intended to diagnose, treat, cure, or prevent any disease."

Also, manufacturers are expected to follow certain good manufacturing practices (GMPs) to ensure that dietary supplements are processed consistently and meet quality standards. Requirements for GMPs went into effect in 2008 for large manufacturers and are being phased in for small manufacturers through 2010.

Once a dietary supplement is on the market, the FDA monitors safety and product information, such as label claims and package inserts. If it finds a product to be unsafe, it can take action against the manufacturer and/or distributor and may issue a warning or require that the product be removed from the marketplace. The Federal Trade Commission (FTC) is responsible for regulating product advertising; it requires that all information be truthful and not misleading.

The federal government has taken legal action against a number of dietary supplement promoters or Web sites that promote or sell dietary supplements because they have made false or deceptive statements about their products or because marketed products have proven to be unsafe.

28. What is the main idea of the passage?
    A. Manufacturers of dietary supplements have to follow good manufacturing practices.
    B. The FDA has a special program for regulating dietary supplements.
    C. The federal government prosecutes those who mislead the general public.
    D. The FDA is part of the federal government.

29. Which statement is *not* a detail from the passage?
    A. Promoters of dietary supplements can make any claims that are supported by research.
    B. GMP requirements for large manufacturers went into effect in 2008.
    C. Product advertising is regulated by the FTC.
    D. The FDA does not monitor products after they enter the market.

30. What is the meaning of the phrase *phased in* as it is used in the third paragraph?
    A. stunned into silence
    B. confused
    C. implemented in stages
    D. legalized

31. What is the meaning of the word *deceptive* as it is used in the fifth paragraph?
    A. misleading
    B. malicious
    C. illegal
    D. irritating

Questions 32 to 35 pertain to the following passage:
    Anemia is a condition in which there is an abnormally low number of red blood cells (RBCs). This condition also can occur if the RBCs don't contain enough hemoglobin, the iron-rich protein that makes the blood red. Hemoglobin helps RBCs carry oxygen from the lungs to the rest of the body.

    Anemia can be accompanied by low numbers of RBCs, white blood cells (WBCs), and platelets. Red blood cells are disc-shaped and look like doughnuts without holes in the center. They carry oxygen and remove carbon dioxide (a waste product) from your body. These cells are made in the bone marrow and live for about 120 days in the bloodstream. Platelets and WBCs also are made in the bone marrow. White blood cells help fight infection. Platelets stick together to seal small cuts or breaks on the blood vessel walls and to stop bleeding.

If you are anemic, your body doesn't get enough oxygenated blood. As a result, you may feel tired or have other symptoms. Severe or long-lasting anemia can damage the heart, brain, and other organs of the body. Very severe anemia may even cause death.

Anemia has three main causes: blood loss, lack of RBC production, or high rates of RBC destruction. Many types of anemia are mild, brief, and easily treated. Some types can be prevented with a healthy diet or treated with dietary supplements. However, certain types of anemia may be severe, long lasting, and life threatening if not diagnosed and treated.

If you have the signs or symptoms of anemia, you should see your doctor to find out whether you have the condition. Treatment will depend on the cause and severity of the anemia.

32. What is the main idea of the passage?
    A. Anemia presents in a number of forms.
    B. Anemia is a potentially dangerous condition characterized by low numbers of RBCs.
    C. Anemia is a deficiency of WBCs and platelets.
    D. Anemia is a treatable condition.

33. Which statement is *not* a detail from the passage?
    A. There are different methods for treating anemia.
    B. Red blood cells remove carbon dioxide from the body.
    C. Platelets are made in the bone marrow.
    D. Anemia is rarely caused by blood loss.

34. What is the meaning of the word *oxygenated* as it is used in the third paragraph?
    A. containing low amounts of oxygen
    B. containing no oxygen
    C. consisting entirely of oxygen
    D. containing high amounts of oxygen

35. What is the meaning of the word *severity* as it is used in the fifth paragraph?
    A. seriousness
    B. disconnectedness
    C. truth
    D. swiftness

Questions 36 to 39 pertain to the following passage :
    Contrary to previous reports, drinking four or more cups of coffee a day does not put women at risk of rheumatoid arthritis (RA), according to a new study partially funded by the National Institute of Arthritis and Musculoskeletal and Skin Diseases (NIAMS). The study concluded that there is little evidence to support a connection between consuming coffee or tea and the risk of RA among women.

    Rheumatoid arthritis is an inflammatory autoimmune disease that affects the joints. It results in pain, stiffness, swelling, joint damage, and loss of function. Inflammation most often affects the hands and feet and tends to be symmetrical. About one percent of the U.S. population has rheumatoid arthritis.

    Elizabeth W. Karlson, M.D., and her colleagues at HarvardMedicalSchool and Brigham and Women's Hospital in Boston, Massachusetts, used the Nurses' Health Study, a long-term investigation of nurses' diseases, lifestyles, and health practices, to examine possible links between caffeinated beverages and RA risk. The researchers were able to follow up more than 90 percent of the original pool of 83,124 participants who answered a 1980 food frequency questionnaire, and no links were found. They also considered changes in diet and habits over a prolonged period of time, and when the results were adjusted for other factors, such as cigarette smoking, alcohol consumption, and oral contraceptive use, the outcome still showed no relationship between caffeine consumption and risk of RA. Previous research had suggested an association between consuming coffee or tea and RA risk. According to Dr. Karlson, the data supporting that conclusion were inconsistent. Because the information in the older studies was collected at only one time, she says, consideration was not given to the other factors associated with RA, such as cigarette smoking and changes in diet and lifestyle over a follow-up period. The new study presents a more accurate picture of caffeine and RA risk.

36. What is the main idea of the passage?
    A. In the past, doctors have cautioned older women to avoid caffeinated beverages.
    B. Rheumatoid arthritis affects the joints of older women.
    C. A recent study found no link between caffeine consumption and RA among women.
    D. Cigarette smoking increases the incidence of RA.

37. Which statement is *not* a detail from the passage?
    A. Alcohol consumption is linked with RA.
    B. The original data for the study came from a 1980 questionnaire.
    C. Rheumatoid arthritis most often affects the hands and feet.
    D. This study included tens of thousands of participants.

38. What is the meaning of the word *symmetrical* as it is used in the second paragraph?
    A. affecting both sides of the body in corresponding fashion
    B. impossible to treat
    C. sensitive to the touch
    D. asymptomatic

39. What is the author's primary purpose in writing the essay?
    A. to entertain
    B. to inform
    C. to analyze
    D. to persuade

Questions 40 to 43 refer to the following passage:
    Exercise is vital at every age for healthy bones. Not only does exercise improve bone health, but it also increases muscle strength, coordination, and balance, and it leads to better overall health. Exercise is especially important for preventing and treating osteoporosis. Like muscle, bone is living tissue that responds to exercise by becoming stronger. Young women and men who exercise regularly generally achieve greater peak bone mass (maximum bone density and strength) than those who do not. For most people, bone mass peaks during the third decade of life. After that time, we can begin to lose bone. Women and men older than age 20 can help prevent bone loss with regular exercise. Exercise maintains muscle strength, coordination, and balance, which in turn prevent falls and related fractures. This is especially important for older adults and people with osteoporosis. Weight-bearing exercise is the best kind of exercise for bones, which forces the muscle to work against gravity. Some examples of weight-bearing exercises are weight training, walking, hiking, jogging, climbing stairs, tennis, and dancing. Swimming and bicycling, on the other hand, are not weight-bearing exercises. Although these activities help build and maintain strong muscles and have excellent cardiovascular benefits, they are not the best exercise for bones.

40. What is the main idea of the passage?
    A. Weight-bearing exercise is the best for bones.
    B. Exercise increases balance.
    C. Exercise improves bone health.
    D. Women benefit from regular exercise more than men.

41. What is the meaning of the word *vital* as it is used in the first paragraph?
    A. deadly
    B. important
    C. rejected
    D. nourishing

42. Which statement is *not* a detail from the passage?
    A. Tennis is a form of weight-bearing exercise.
    B. Most people reach peak bone mass in their twenties.
    C. Swimming is not good for the bones.
    D. Bone is a living tissue.

43. What is the meaning of the word *fractures* as it is used in the second paragraph?
    A. breaks
    B. agreements
    C. tiffs
    D. fevers

Questions 44 to 47 pertain to the following passage :

Searching for medical information can be confusing, especially for first-timers. However, if you are patient and stick to it, you can find a wealth of information. Your community library is a good place to start your search for medical information. Before going to the library, you may find it helpful to make a list of topics you want information about and questions you have. Your list of topics and questions will make it easier for the librarian to direct you to the best resources.

Many community libraries have a collection of basic medical references. These references may include medical dictionaries or encyclopedias, drug information handbooks, basic medical and nursing textbooks, and directories of physicians and medical specialists (listings of doctors). You may also find magazine articles on a certain topic. Look in the Reader's Guide to Periodical Literature for articles on health and medicine from consumer magazines.

Infotrac, a CD-ROM computer database available at libraries or on the Web, indexes hundreds of popular magazines and newspapers, as well as medical journals such as the Journal of the American Medical Association and New England Journal of Medicine. Your library may also carry searchable computer databases of medical journal articles, including MEDLINE/PubMed or the Cumulative Index to Nursing and Allied Health Literature. Many of the databases or indexes have abstracts that provide a summary of each journal article. Although most community libraries don't have a large collection of medical and nursing journals, your librarian may be able to get copies of the articles you want. Interlibrary loans allow your librarian to request a copy of an article from a library that carries that particular medical journal. Your library may charge a fee for this service. Articles published in medical journals can be technical, but they may be the most current source of information on medical topics.

44. What is the main idea of the passage?
    A. Infotrac is a useful source of information.
    B. The community library offers numerous resources for medical information.
    C. Searching for medical information can be confusing.
    D. There is no reason to prepare a list of topics before visiting the library.

45. What is the meaning of the word *popular* as it is used in the third paragraph?
    A. complicated
    B. old-fashioned
    C. beloved
    D. for the general public

46. Which statement is *not* a detail from the passage?
    A. Abstracts summarize the information in an article.
    B. Having a prepared list of questions enables the librarian to serve you better.
    C. Infotrac is a database on CD-ROM.
    D. The articles in popular magazines can be hard to understand.

47. What is the meaning of the word *technical* as it is used in the fourth paragraph?
    A. requiring expert knowledge
    B. incomplete
    C. foreign
    D. plagiarized

Section 2. Vocabulary and General Knowledge

Number of Questions: **50**	
Time Limit: **50 Minutes**	

1. What is the meaning of the word *prognosis*?
   A. forecast
   B. description
   C. outline
   D. schedule

2. What is the name for any substance that stimulates the production of antibodies?
   A. collagen
   B. hemoglobin
   C. lymph
   D. antigen

3. What is the best definition for the word *abstain*?
   A. offend
   B. retrain
   C. to refrain from
   D. defenestrate

4. Select the meaning of the underlined word in this sentence:
Jerry held out hope for recovery, in spite of the <u>ominous</u> results from the lab.
   A. threatening
   B. emboldening
   C. destructive
   D. insightful

5. What is the meaning of the word *incidence*?
   A. random events
   B. sterility
   C. autonomy
   D. rate of occurrence

6. Select the word that means "water loving."
   A. homologous
   B. hydrophilia
   C. dipsomaniac
   D. hydrated

7. Select the meaning of the underlined word in this sentence:
The <u>occluded</u> artery posed a significant threat to the long-term health of the patient.
   A. closed
   B. deformed
   C. enlarged
   D. engorged

8. What is the best description for the word *potent*?
    A. frantic
    B. determined
    C. feverish
    D. powerful

9. Select the meaning of the underlined word in this sentence:
The doctors were less concerned with Bill's respiration than with the <u>precipitous</u> rise in his blood pressure.
    A. detached
    B. sordid
    C. encompassed
    D. steep

10. Select the meaning of the underlined word in this sentence:
It is <u>vital</u> for the victim of a serious accident to receive medical attention immediately.
    A. recommended
    B. discouraged
    C. essential
    D. sufficient

11. What is the best description for the word *insidious*?
    A. stealthy
    B. deadly
    C. collapsed
    D. new

12. Select the word that means "take into the body."
    A. congest
    B. ingest
    C. collect
    D. suppress

13. What is the meaning of the word *proscribe*?
    A. anticipate
    B. prevent
    C. defeat
    D. forbid

14. Select the meaning of the underlined word in this sentence.
Wracked by abdominal pain, the victim of food poisoning moaned and rubbed his <u>distended</u> belly.
    A. concave
    B. sore
    C. swollen
    D. empty

15. Select the meaning of the underlined word in this sentence:
Despite the absence of <u>overt</u> signs, Dr. Harris suspected that Alicia might be suffering from the flu.
    A. concealed
    B. apparent
    C. expert
    D. delectable

16. Select the word that means "something added to resolve a deficiency or obtain completion."
    A. supplement
    B. complement
    C. detriment
    D. acumen

17. Select the word that means "a violent seizure."
    A. revelation
    B. nutrient
    C. contraption
    D. paroxysm

18. What is the meaning of *carnivore*?
    A. hungry
    B. meat eating
    C. infected
    D. demented

19. What is the meaning of *belligerent*?
    A. retired
    B. sardonic
    C. pugnacious
    D. acclimated

20. Select the word that means "on both sides."
    A. bilateral
    B. insufficient
    C. bicuspid
    D. congruent

21. Select the meaning of the underlined word in this sentence:
The medication should only be taken if the old symptoms <u>recur</u>.
    A. occur again
    B. survive
    C. collect
    D. desist

22. Select the word that means "likely to change."
    A. venereal
    B. motile
    C. labile
    D. entrail

23. What is the best description for the word *flaccid*?
    A. defended
    B. limp
    C. slender
    D. outdated

24. Select the word that means "both male and female."
    A. monozygotic
    B. heterogeneous
    C. homologous
    D. androgynous

25. What is the meaning of *terrestrial*?
    A. alien
    B. earthly
    C. foreign
    D. domestic

26. Select the word that means "improper or unfortunate."
    A. allocated
    B. untoward
    C. flaccid
    D. dilated

27. Select the meaning of the underlined word in this sentence:
At first, Gerald suspected that he had caught the disease at the office; later, though, he concluded that it was <u>endogenous</u>.
    A. contagious
    B. painful to the touch
    C. continuous
    D. growing from within

28. What is the meaning of *symptom*?
    A. result
    B. indication
    C. side effect
    D. precondition

29. Select the word that means "intrusive."
    A. convulsive
    B. destructive
    C. invasive
    D. connective

30. What is the meaning of *parameter*?
    A. guideline
    B. standard
    C. manual
    D. variable

31. Select the word that means "empty."
    A. holistic
    B. void
    C. concrete
    D. maladjusted

32. Select the meaning of the underlined word in this sentence:
Though chemotherapy had sent her cancer into remission, Glenda remained <u>lethargic</u> and depressed.
    A. nauseous
    B. sluggish
    C. contagious
    D. elated

33. Select the word that means "offsetting."
    A. compensatory
    B. defensive
    C. untoward
    D. confused

34. Select the word that means "degeneration or wasting away."
    A. dystrophy
    B. entropy
    C. atrophy
    D. apathy

35. What is the best description for the word *discrete*?
    A. calm
    B. subtle
    C. hidden
    D. separate

36. Select the meaning of the underlined word in this sentence:
In order to minimize scarring, the nurse reused the <u>site</u> of the previous injection.
    A. syringe
    B. location
    C. artery
    D. hole

37. Select the meaning of the underlined word in this sentence:
As a veteran of many flu seasons, the nurse knew how to minimize her <u>exposure</u> to the disease.
    A. laying open
    B. prohibition
    C. connection
    D. dislike

38. What is the meaning of *exacerbate*?
    A. implicate
    B. aggravate
    C. heal
    D. decondition

39. Select the word that means "nerve cell."
    A. neutron
    B. nucleus
    C. neuron
    D. neutral

40. Select the word that means "unfavorable."
    A. liberated
    B. adverse
    C. convenient
    D. occluded

41. Select the meaning of the underlined word in this sentence:
Dr. Grant ignored Mary's particular symptoms, instead administering a <u>holistic</u> treatment for her condition.
    A. insensitive
    B. ignorant
    C. specialized
    D. concerned with the whole rather than the parts

42. What is the best description for the word *suppress*?
    A. stop
    B. push up
    C. release
    D. strain

43. Select the word that means "about to happen."
    A. depending
    B. offending
    C. suspending
    D. impending

44. Select the meaning of the underlined word in this sentence:
The dermatologist was struck by the <u>symmetric</u> patterns of scarring on the patient's back.
    A. scabbed
    B. painful to the touch
    C. occurring in corresponding parts at the same time
    D. geometric

45. Select the word that means "open."
    A. inverted
    B. patent
    C. convent
    D. converted

46. Select the meaning of the underlined word in this sentence:
Despite an increase in the <u>volume</u> of his urine, the patient still reported bloating.
    A. quality
    B. length
    C. quantity
    D. loudness

47. What is the meaning of *repugnant*?
    A. destructive
    B. selective
    C. collective
    D. offensive

48. Select the word that means "enlarge."
    A. dilate
    B. protrude
    C. confuse
    D. occlude

49. What is the best description for the word *intact*?
    A. collapsed
    B. disconnected
    C. unbroken
    D. free

50. Select the word that means "the ability to enter, contact, or approach."
    A. ingress
    B. excess
    C. access
    D. success

Section 3. Grammar

Number of Questions: **50**	
Time Limit: **50 Minutes**	

1. Which word is *not* spelled correctly in the context of the following sentence?
Dr. Vargas was surprised that the prescription had effected Ron's fatigue so dramatically.
   A. surprised
   B. prescription
   C. effected
   D. fatigue

2. Select the word that makes this sentence grammatically correct:
Is the new student coming out to lunch with ____?
   A. we
   B. our
   C. us
   D. they

3. Select the word or phrase that makes this sentence grammatically correct:
____ picking up groceries one of the things you are supposed to do?
   A. Is
   B. Am
   C. Is it
   D. Are

4. Select the word that makes the following sentence grammatically correct.
These days, you can't ____ learning how to use a computer.
   A. not
   B. cvading
   C. despite
   D. avoid

5. Which word is *not* spelled correctly in the context of the following sentence?
The climate hear is inappropriate for snow sports such as skiing.
   A. climate
   B. hear
   C. inappropriate
   D. skiing

6. Select the word or phrase that makes the following sentence grammatically correct.
____ screaming took the shopkeeper by surprise.
   A. We
   B. They
   C. Them
   D. Our

7. Select the word or phrase that makes the following sentence grammatically correct.
Why did we ____ try so hard?
    A. has to
    B. haven't
    C. had to
    D. have to

8. Select the word that makes the following sentence grammatically correct.
Tracey wore her hair in a French braid, ____ was the style at the time.
    A. among
    B. it
    C. that
    D. which

9. Select the phrase that makes the following sentence grammatically correct.
Working _____ the mission of the entire committee.
    A. to peace is
    B. toward peace was
    C. to peace was
    D. toward peace am

10. Select the phrase that makes the following sentence grammatically correct.
Janet called her _____ run after a squirrel.
    A. dog, who had
    B. dog that had
    C. dog, that had
    D. dog who had

11. Select the correct word for the blank in the following sentence.
After completing the intense surgery, Dr. Capra needed a long ____.
    A. brake
    B. break
    C. brink
    D. broke

12. Select the correct word for the blank in the following sentence.
The other day, Stan ____ reviewing his class notes in preparation for the final exam.
    A. begins
    B. begun
    C. begin
    D. began

13. Select the word or phrase that makes the following sentence grammatically correct.
It makes sense to maintain your current prescriptions, ____ they have worked so well in the past.
    A. although
    B. despite that
    C. since
    D. but

14. Select the word or phrase that makes the following sentence grammatically correct.
It seems like his blood pressure ___ every week.
    A. rises
    B. raises
    C. raise
    D. rise

15. Select the word or phrase that makes the following sentence correct.
____ their similar training, the two professionals drew radically different conclusions.
    A. Because of
    B. Among
    C. Despite
    D. Now that

16. Select the word or phrase that makes the following sentence grammatically correct.
Each of the two European capitals ____ named after a famous leader.
    A. are
    B. am
    C. as
    D. is

17. Which word is *not* used correctly in the context of the following sentence?
Before you walk any further, beware of the approaching traffic.
    A. before
    B. further
    C. beware
    D. approaching

18. What word is used incorrectly in the following sentence?
The little boy sat the red block atop the stack.
    A. little
    B. sat
    C. atop
    D. stack

19. Select the word or phrase that makes the following sentence grammatically correct.
Even though she was new, Lauren knew that ___ the patient's name would be an ethical violation.
    A. divulge
    B. to divulge
    C. to divulging
    D. divulged

20. Select the word or phrase that makes the following sentence grammatically correct.
The attendant looked ____ at everything related to the problem.
    A. close
    B. closet
    C. closely
    D. closedly

21. What word or phrase is used incorrectly in the following sentence?
Henry intuitively understood the doctor's illusion to his long-term depression.
  A. intuitively
  B. illusion
  C. long-term
  D. depression

22. Select the correct word for the blank in the following sentence.
If you want to join the club, you ____ contact the coach by Thursday.
  A. would
  B. should
  C. did
  D. have

23. Select the word that makes the following sentence grammatically correct.
Andy has ____ up a law practice of his own.
  A. seat
  B. set
  C. sit
  D. sat

24. Select the word or phrase that makes the following sentence grammatically correct.
He decided to buy a large coal furnace because he felt it would be _____ than a woodstove.
  A. more efficient
  B. efficienter
  C. more efficienter
  D. efficiency

25. What word is used incorrectly in the following sentence?
It is amazing how many soccer players has developed knee problems over the years.
  A. many
  B. players
  C. has
  D. developed

26. Select the word that makes the following sentence grammatically correct.
She asked __ to take her around the corner to the drugstore.
  A. him
  B. his
  C. he
  D. his'

27. Select the word or phrase that makes the following sentence grammatically correct.
Felix was pleased ____ the progress he had made in his program.
  A. among
  B. with
  C. regards
  D. besides

28. Select the word or phrase that makes the following sentence grammatically correct.
After waking up, Dean eyed the cheesecake _____.
    A. hungry
    B. hungriest
    C. hungrily
    D. more hungry

29. Which word is *not* used correctly in the context of the following sentence?
After ringing up the nails, the cashier handed Nedra her recipe and change.
    A. ringing
    B. cashier
    C. recipe
    D. change

30. Select the correct word for the blank in the following sentence.
Sharon felt ____ about how her speech had gone.
    A. well
    B. good
    C. finely
    D. happily

31. What word is used incorrectly in the following sentence?
Brendan spent the day lying a brick foundation on the site.
    A. site
    B. on
    C. spent
    D. lying

32. Select the word or phrase that makes this sentence grammatically correct:
Children _____ obey their parents tend to do better in school.
    A. who
    B. which
    C. should
    D. to

33. Select the word or phrase that makes this sentence grammatically correct:
The development committee ____ a bargain with the city planners.
    A. striked
    B. stroke
    C. struck
    D. strike

34. Select the word or phrase that makes this sentence grammatically correct:
A child is not yet old enough to know what is healthy for _____.
    A. him or her
    B. them
    C. it
    D. she or he

35. Select the word or phrase that makes this sentence grammatically correct:
Theo was in great shape; he _____ all the way back to the pier.
    A. swam
    B. swimmed
    C. swum
    D. swim

36. Select the phrase that makes this sentence grammatically correct:
_____ went to the movies after having dinner at Lenny's.
    A. Her and I
    B. Her and me
    C. She and I
    D. She and me

37. Select the word or phrase that makes this sentence grammatically correct:
Before turning in, Brian made sure to ____ the alarm clock.
    A. sat
    B. sit
    C. set
    D. setted

38. What word is used incorrectly in the following sentence?
The dashboard shaked as he revved the engine.
    A. dashboard
    B. shaked
    C. as
    D. revved

39. Select the word or phrase that makes this sentence grammatically correct:
_____ way he looked, Ted saw people milling about.
    A. Moreover
    B. Whichever
    C. Whomever
    D. Whether

40. Select the correct word for the blank in the following sentence.
The buried treasure had ____ there for centuries.
    A. laid
    B. layed
    C. lain
    D. laint

41. Select the word that makes this sentence grammatically correct:
In order to serve each patient better, the clinic decided to see ____ patients overall.
    A. less
    B. fewer
    C. lesser
    D. few

42. Select the word or phrase that makes this sentence grammatically correct:
It wasn't until ____ the interview that Kim realized she had forgotten her list of questions.
  A. despite
  B. after
  C. among
  D. between

43. Which word is used incorrectly in the following sentence?
The video store is on the way, so we should stop by and rent one.
  A. video
  B. way
  C. by
  D. one

44. Select the word that makes the following sentence grammatically correct.
____ are the best eye doctors in this county?
  A. Who
  B. Which
  C. Whom
  D. What

45. Select the word that makes this sentence grammatically correct:
While he was an apprentice, Steve ____ a great deal of time in the studio.
  A. spends
  B. spent
  C. spended
  D. spend

46. Select the word that correctly completes the following sentence.
The intern was surprised by the _____ of pain he was in after his first day of work.
  A. amount
  B. frequency
  C. number
  D. amplitude

47. What word is used incorrectly in the following sentence?
Whoever wrote the letter forgot to sign their name.
  A. Whoever
  B. wrote
  C. their
  D. name

48. Select the word or phrase that makes this sentence grammatically correct:
The child's fever was ___ high for him to lie comfortably in bed.
  A. to
  B. much
  C. too
  D. more

49. Select the word or phrase that makes the following sentence grammatically correct.
Sometimes, the condition _____ with an unusual symptom—vertigo.
   A. presence
   B. presents
   C. present
   D. prescience

50. Which word is *not* used correctly in the context of the following sentence?
There is no real distinction among the two treatment protocols recommended online.
   A. real
   B. among
   C. protocols
   D. online

Section 4. Mathematics

Number of Questions: **50**
Time Limit: **50 Minutes**

1. 474 + 2038 =
   A. 2512
   B. 2412
   C. 2521
   D. 2502

2. 32,788 + 1693 =
   A. 33,481
   B. 32,383
   C. 34,481
   D. 36,481

3. 3703 – 1849 =
   A. 1954
   B. 1854
   C. 1974
   D. 1794

4. 4790 – 2974 =
   A. 1816
   B. 1917
   C. 2109
   D. 1779

5. 229 × 738 =
   A. 161,622
   B. 167,670
   C. 169,002
   D. 171,451

6. 356 × 808 =
   A. 274,892
   B. 278,210
   C. 283,788
   D. 287,648

7. Round to the nearest whole number: 435 ÷ 7 =
   A. 16
   B. 62
   C. 74
   D. 86

8. Round to the nearest whole number: 4748 ÷ 12 =
   A. 372
   B. 384
   C. 396
   D. 412

3 HESI Admission Assessment Practice Tests

9. Report all decimal places: 3.7 + 7.289 + 4 =
   A. 14.989
   B. 5.226
   C. 15.0
   D. 15.07

10. 4.934 + 7.1 + 9.08 =
   A. 21.114
   B. 21.042
   C. 20.214
   D. 59.13

11. 27 – 3.54 =
   A. 24.56
   B. 23.46
   C. 33.3
   D. 24.54

12. 28.19 – 9 =
   A. 28.1
   B. 18.19
   C. 27.29
   D. 19.19

13. Karen goes to the grocery store with $40. She buys a carton of milk for $1.85, a loaf of bread for $3.20, and a bunch of bananas for $3.05. How much money does she have left?
   A. $30.95
   B. $31.90
   C. $32.10
   D. $34.95

14. Round your answer to the tenths place:0.088 × 277.9 =
   A. 21.90
   B. 2.5
   C. 24.5
   D. 24.46

15. Round your answer to the hundredths place:28 ÷ 0.6 =
   A. 46.67
   B. 0.021
   C. 17.50
   D. 16.8

16. Roger's car gets an average of 25 miles per gallon. If his gas tank holds 16 gallons, about how far can he drive on a full tank?
   A. 41 miles
   B. 100 miles
   C. 320 miles
   D. 400 miles

17. Express the answer in simplest form: $\dfrac{3}{8} + \dfrac{2}{8} =$

    A. $\dfrac{1}{8}$

    B. $\dfrac{1}{2}$

    C. $\dfrac{5}{8}$

    D. $\dfrac{5}{16}$

18. Express the answer in simplest form: $\dfrac{2}{3} + \dfrac{2}{7} =$

    A. $\dfrac{20}{21}$

    B. $\dfrac{4}{10}$

    C. $\dfrac{4}{21}$

    D. $\dfrac{2}{5}$

19. Present the sum as a mixed number in simplest form: $1\dfrac{1}{2} + \dfrac{12}{9} =$

    A. $2\dfrac{3}{5}$

    B. $1\dfrac{3}{4}$

    C. $3\dfrac{1}{3}$

    D. $2\dfrac{5}{6}$

20. Aaron worked $2\dfrac{1}{2}$ hours on Monday, $3\dfrac{3}{4}$ hours on Tuesday, and $7\dfrac{2}{3}$ hours on Thursday. How many hours did he work in all?

    A. $10\dfrac{5}{6}$

    B. $12\dfrac{1}{2}$

    C. $13\dfrac{1}{4}$

    D. $13\dfrac{11}{12}$

21. Express the answer in simplest form: $\dfrac{23}{24} - \dfrac{11}{24} =$

    A. $\dfrac{11}{23}$

    B. $\dfrac{1}{2}$

    C. $\dfrac{2}{3}$

    D. $\dfrac{12}{24}$

22. Express the answer in simplest form: $3\dfrac{4}{7} - 2\dfrac{3}{14} =$

    A. $2\dfrac{3}{14}$

    B. $1\dfrac{1}{14}$

    C. $1\dfrac{5}{14}$

    D. $2\dfrac{3}{7}$

23. Express the answer in simplest form: Dean has brown, white, and black socks. One-third of his socks are white; one-sixth of his socks are black. How many of his socks are brown?

    A. $\dfrac{1}{3}$

    B. $\dfrac{2}{6}$

    C. $\dfrac{1}{2}$

    D. $\dfrac{3}{4}$

24. Express the answer in simplest form: A recipe calls for $1\dfrac{1}{2}$ cups sugar, $3\dfrac{2}{3}$ cups flour, and $\dfrac{2}{3}$ cup milk. If you want to double the recipe, what will be the total amount of cups of ingredients required?

    A. $11\dfrac{2}{3}$

    B. 8

    C. $12\dfrac{1}{6}$

    D. $6\dfrac{2}{3}$

25. Express your answer as a mixed number in simplest form: $4\dfrac{1}{3} \times \dfrac{2}{7} =$

   A. $6\dfrac{1}{3}$

   B. $3\dfrac{7}{10}$

   C. $\dfrac{8}{21}$

   D. $1\dfrac{5}{21}$

26. Express the answer as a mixed number or fraction in simplest form: $2\dfrac{3}{9} \times \dfrac{1}{3} =$

   A. $\dfrac{7}{8}$

   B. $2\dfrac{3}{7}$

   C. $\dfrac{12}{27}$

   D. $\dfrac{7}{9}$

27. Express the answer as a mixed number or fraction in simplest form: $\dfrac{5}{8} \div \dfrac{1}{5} =$

   A. $\dfrac{1}{8}$

   B. $2\dfrac{3}{4}$

   C. $3\dfrac{1}{3}$

   D. $3\dfrac{1}{8}$

28. Express the answer as a mixed number or fraction in simplest form: $\dfrac{2}{7} \div \dfrac{1}{6} =$

   A. $\dfrac{1}{21}$

   B. $2\dfrac{1}{12}$

   C. $1\dfrac{3}{4}$

   D. $1\dfrac{5}{7}$

29. Round to the nearest whole number:Bill got $\frac{7}{9}$ of the answers right on his chemistry test. On a scale of 1 to 100, what numerical grade would he receive?

    A. 77

    B. 78

    C. 79

    D. 80

30. Round to the hundredths place.Change the fraction to a decimal: $\frac{7}{8} =$

    A. 0.88

    B. 0.92

    C. 0.84

    D. 0.78

31. Round to the hundredths place.Change the fraction to a decimal: $4\frac{3}{7} =$

    A. 4.37

    B. 4.43

    C. 4.56

    D. 4.78

32. Change the decimal to the simplest equivalent proper fraction:3.78 =

    A. $3\frac{3}{4}$

    B. $3\frac{7}{8}$

    C. $3\frac{39}{50}$

    D. $3\frac{78}{100}$

33. Change the decimal to the simplest equivalent proper fraction:0.07 =

    A. $\frac{7}{10}$

    B. $\frac{0.07}{10}$

    C. $\frac{7}{100}$

    D. $\frac{70}{100}$

34. Change the decimal to the simplest equivalent proper fraction:2.80 =

A. $\dfrac{2.8}{10}$

B. $2\dfrac{8}{10}$

C. $\dfrac{0.28}{1}$

D. $2\dfrac{4}{5}$

35. Change the fraction to the simplest possible ratio: $\dfrac{8}{14}$

A. 2:3

B. 4:7

C. 4:6

D. 3:5

36. Two-thirds of the students in Mr. Garcia's class are boys. If there are 27 students in the class, how many of them are girls?

A. 1

B. 9

C. 12

D. 20

37. Solve for x:

3:2 :: 24:x

A. 16

B. 12

C. 2

D. 22

38.Solve for x:

7:42 :: 4:x

A. 12

B. 48

C. 24

D. 16

39. Change the decimal to a percent:0.64 =

A. 0.64%

B. 64%

C. 6.4%

D. 0.064%

40. Change the decimal to a percent:0.000026 =

A. 0.0026%

B. 0.026%

C. 2.6%

D. 26%

41. Change the percent to a decimal:38% =
    A. 3.8
    B. 0.038
    C. 38.0
    D. 0.38

42. Change the percent to a decimal:17.6% =
    A. 17.6
    B. 1.76
    C. 0.176
    D. 0.0176

43. Change the percent to a decimal:126% =
    A. 126.0
    B. 0.0126
    C. 0.126
    D. 1.26

44. Round to the nearest whole number.Change the fraction to a percent: $\dfrac{2}{9}$ =

    A. 20%
    B. 21%
    C. 22%
    D. 23%

45. Round to the nearest whole number.Change the fraction to a percent: $\dfrac{9}{13}$ =

    A. 33%
    B. 69%
    C. 72%
    D. 78%

46. Round to the nearest whole number:What is 17 out of 68, as a percent?
    A. 17%
    B. 25%
    C. 32%
    D. 68%

47. Round to the nearest percentage point:Gerald made 13 out of the 22 shots he took in the basketball game. What was his shooting percentage?
    A. 13%
    B. 22%
    C. 59%
    D. 67%

48. Round to the nearest whole number:What is 18% of 600?
    A. 108
    B. 76
    C. 254
    D. 176

49. Round to the tenths place:What is 6.4% of 32?
    A. 1.8
    B. 2.1
    C. 2.6
    D. 2.0

50. What is the numerical value of the Roman number XVII?
    A. 22
    B. 17
    C. 48
    D. 57

| Section 5. Biology | Number of Questions: **25** |
| | Time Limit: **25 Minutes** |

1. If an organism is *AaBb*, which of the following combinations in the gametes is impossible?
   A. AB
   B. aa
   C. aB
   D. Ab

2. What is the typical result of mitosis in humans?
   A. two diploid cells
   B. two haploid cells
   C. four diploid cells
   D. four haploid cells

3. How does water affect the temperature of a living thing?
   A. Water increases temperature.
   B. Water keeps temperature stable.
   C. Water decreases temperature.
   D. Water does not affect temperature.

4. Which of the following is *not* a product of the Krebs cycle?
   A. carbon dioxide
   B. oxygen
   C. adenosine triphosphate (ATP)
   D. energy carriers

5. What kind of bond connects sugar and phosphate in DNA?
   A. hydrogen
   B. ionic
   C. covalent
   D. overt

6. What is the second part of an organism's scientific name?
   A. species
   B. phylum
   C. population
   D. kingdom

7. How are lipids different than other organic molecules?
   A. They are indivisible.
   B. They are not water soluble.
   C. They contain zinc.
   D. They form long proteins.

8. Which of the following is *not* a steroid?
   A. cholesterol
   B. estrogen
   C. testosterone
   D. hemoglobin

9. Which of the following properties is responsible for the passage of water through a plant?
   A. cohesion
   B. adhesion
   C. osmosis
   D. evaporation

10. Which hormone is produced by the pineal gland?
   A. insulin
   B. testosterone
   C. melatonin
   D. epinephrine

11. What is the name of the organelle that organizes protein synthesis?
   A. mitochondrion
   B. nucleus
   C. ribosome
   D. vacuole

12. During which phase is the chromosome number reduced from diploid to haploid?
   A. S phase
   B. interphase
   C. mitosis
   D. meiosis I

13. What is the name for a cell that does *not* contain a nucleus?
   A. eukaryote
   B. bacteria
   C. prokaryote
   D. cancer

14. What is the name for the physical presentation of an organism's genes?
   A. phenotype
   B. species
   C. phylum
   D. genotype

15. Which of the following forms of water is the densest?
   A. liquid
   B. steam
   C. ice
   D. All forms of water have the same density.

16. What is the longest phase in the life of a cell?
   A. prophase
   B. interphase
   C. anaphase
   D. metaphase

17. Which of the following is *not* found within a bacterial cell?
    A. mitochondria
    B. DNA
    C. vesicles
    D. ribosome

18. Which of the following is a protein?
    A. cellulose
    B. hemoglobin
    C. estrogen
    D. ATP

19. Which of the following structures is *not* involved in translation?
    A. tRNA
    B. mRNA
    C. ribosome
    D. DNA

20. Which of the following is necessary for cell diffusion?
    A. water
    B. membrane
    C. ATP
    D. gradient

21. How many different types of nucleotides are there in DNA?
    A. one
    B. two
    C. four
    D. eight

22. Which of the following cell types has no nucleus?
    A. platelet
    B. red blood cell
    C. white blood cell
    D. phagocyte

23. Which part of aerobic respiration uses oxygen?
    A. osmosis
    B. Krebs cycle
    C. glycolysis
    D. electron transport system

24. Which of the following is the most general taxonomic category?
    A. kingdom
    B. phylum
    C. genus
    D. order

25. What is the name of the process by which a bacterial cell splits into two new cells?
    A. mitosis
    B. meiosis
    C. replication
    D. fission

Section 6. Chemistry

Number of Questions: **25**	
Time Limit: **25 Minutes**	

1. Which of the following substances allows for the fastest diffusion?
    A. gas
    B. solid
    C. liquid
    D. plasma

2. What is the oxidation number of hydrogen in CaH_2?
    A. +1
    B. −1
    C. 0
    D. +2

3. Which of the following does *not* exist as a diatomic molecule?
    A. boron
    B. fluorine
    C. oxygen
    D. nitrogen

4. What is another name for aqueous HI?
    A. hydroiodate acid
    B. hydrogen monoiodide
    C. hydrogen iodide
    D. hydriodic acid

5. Which of the following could be an empirical formula?
    A. C4H8
    B. C2H6
    C. CH
    D. C3H6

6. What is the name for the reactant that is entirely consumed by the reaction?
    A. limiting reactant
    B. reducing agent
    C. reaction intermediate
    D. reagent

7. What is the name for the horizontal rows of the periodic table?
    A. groups
    B. periods
    C. families
    D. sets

8. What is the mass (in grams) of 7.35 mol water?
    A. 10.7 g
    B. 18 g
    C. 132 g
    D. 180.6 g

9. Which of the following orbitals is the last to fill?
    A. 1s
    B. 3s
    C. 4p
    D. 6s

10. What is the name of the binary molecular compound NO_5?
    A. nitro pentoxide
    B. ammonium pentoxide
    C. nitrogen pentoxide
    D. pentnitrogen oxide

11. What is the mass (in grams) of 1.0 mol oxygen gas?
    A. 12 g
    B. 16 g
    C. 28 g
    D. 32 g

12. Which kind of radiation has no charge?
    A. beta
    B. alpha
    C. delta
    D. gamma

13. What is the name of the state in which forward and reverse chemical reactions are occurring at the same rate?
    A. equilibrium
    B. constancy
    C. stability
    D. toxicity

14. What is 119°K in degrees Celsius?
    A. 32°C
    B. –154°C
    C. 154°C
    D. –32°C

15. What is the SI unit of energy?
    A. ohm
    B. joule
    C. henry
    D. newton

16. What is the name of the device that separates gaseous ions by their mass-to-charge ratio?
    A. mass spectrometer
    B. interferometer
    C. magnetometer
    D. capacitance meter

17. Which material has the smallest specific heat?
    A. water
    B. wood
    C. aluminum
    D. glass

18. What is the name for a reaction in which electrons are transferred from one atom to another?
    A. combustion reaction
    B. synthesis reaction
    C. redox reaction
    D. double-displacement reaction

19. What are van der Waals forces?
    A. the weak forces of attraction between two molecules
    B. the strong forces of attraction between two molecules
    C. hydrogen bonds
    D. conjugal bonds

20. Which of the following gases effuses the fastest?
    A. Cl2
    B. O2
    C. N2
    D. H_2

21. Which of the following elements is *not* involved in many hydrogen bonds?
    A. fluorine
    B. carbon
    C. oxygen
    D. nitrogen

22. What is the mass (in grams) of 0.350 mol copper?
    A. 12.5 g
    B. 14.6 g
    C. 18.5 g
    D. 22.2 g

23. How many d orbitals are there in a d subshell?
    A. 5
    B. 7
    C. 9
    D. 11

24. What is the name for the number of protons in an atom?
    A. atomic identity
    B. atomic mass
    C. atomic weight
    D. atomic number

25. Which of the following elements is an alkali metal?
    A. magnesium
    B. rubidium
    C. hydrogen
    D. chlorine

Section 7. Anatomy and Physiology	Number of Questions: **25**
	Time Limit: **25 Minutes**

1. What is the name of the structure that prevents food from entering the airway?
    A. trachea
    B. esophagus
    C. diaphragm
    D. epiglottis

2. Which substance makes up the pads that provide support between the vertebrae?
    A. bone
    B. cartilage
    C. tendon
    D. fat

3. How many different types of tissue are there in the human body?
    A. four
    B. six
    C. eight
    D. ten

4. What is the name of the outermost layer of skin?
    A. dermis
    B. epidermis
    C. subcutaneous tissue
    D. hypodermis

5. Which hormone stimulates milk production in the breasts during lactation?
    A. norepinephrine
    B. antidiuretic hormone
    C. prolactin
    D. oxytocin

6. Which of the following structures has the lowest blood pressure?
    A. arteries
    B. arteriole
    C. venule
    D. vein

7. Which of the heart chambers is the most muscular?
    A. left atrium
    B. right atrium
    C. left ventricle
    D. right ventricle

8. Which part of the brain interprets sensory information?
   A. cerebrum
   B. hindbrain
   C. cerebellum
   D. medulla oblongata

9. Which of the following proteins is produced by cartilage?
   A. actin
   B. estrogen
   C. collagen
   D. myosin

10. Which component of the nervous system is responsible for lowering the heart rate?
    A. central nervous system
    B. sympathetic nervous system
    C. parasympathetic nervous system
    D. distal nervous system

11. Which type of substance breaks down to form urea?
    A. lipid
    B. protein
    C. carbohydrate
    D. iron

12. What is the name for a joint that can only move in two directions?
    A. hinge
    B. insertion
    C. ball and socket
    D. flange

13. In which of the following muscle types are the filaments arranged in a disorderly manner?
    A. cardiac
    B. smooth
    C. skeletal
    D. rough

14. How much air does an adult inhale in an average breath?
    A. 500 mL
    B. 750 mL
    C. 1000 mL
    D. 1250 mL

15. Which type of cell secretes antibodies?
    A. bacterial cell
    B. viral cell
    C. lymph cell
    D. plasma cells

16. Which force motivates filtration in the kidneys?
    A. osmosis
    B. smooth muscle contraction
    C. peristalsis
    D. blood pressure

17. Which of the following hormones decreases the concentration of blood glucose?
    A. insulin
    B. glucagon
    C. growth hormone
    D. glucocorticoids

18. Which structure controls the hormones secreted by the pituitary gland?
    A. hypothalamus
    B. adrenal gland
    C. testes
    D. pancreas

19. How much of a female's blood volume is composed of red blood cells?
    A. 10%
    B. 25%
    C. 40%
    D. 70%

20. Which type of cholesterol is considered to be the best for health?
    A. LDL
    B. HDL
    C. VLDL
    D. VHDL

21. Where are the vocal cords located?
    A. bronchi
    B. trachea
    C. larynx
    D. epiglottis

22. Where does gas exchange occur in the human body?
    A. alveoli
    B. bronchi
    C. larynx
    D. pharynx

23. Which structure of the nervous system carries action potential in the direction of a synapse?
    A. cell body
    B. axon
    C. neuron
    D. myelin

24. Where is the parathyroid gland located?
   A. neck
   B. back
   C. side
   D. brain

25. What is the name of the process in the lungs by which oxygen is transported from the air to the blood?
   A. osmosis
   B. diffusion
   C. dissipation
   D. reverse osmosis

AnswerExplanations

ReadingComprehensionAnswerKeyandExplanations

1. D: The main idea of this passage is that vaccines help the immune system function properly. Identifying main ideas is one of the key skills tested by the HESI exam. One of the common traps that many test-takers fall into is assuming that the first sentence of the passage will express the main idea. Although this will be true for some passages, often the author will use the first sentence to attract interest or to make an introductory, but not central, point. On this question, if you assume that the first sentence contains the main idea, you will mistakenly choose answer B. Finding the main idea of a passage requires patience and thoroughness; you cannot expect to know the main idea until you have read the entire passage. In this case, a diligent reading will show you that answer choices A, B, and C express details from the passage, but only answer choice D is a comprehensive summary of the author's message.

2. C: This passage does not state that the symptoms of disease will not emerge until the body has learned to fight the disease. The reading comprehension section of the HESI exam will include several questions that require you to identify details from a passage. The typical structure of these questions is to ask you to identify the answer choice that contains a detail not included in the passage. This question structure makes your work a little more difficult, because it requires you to confirm that the other three details are in the passage. In this question, the details expressed in answer choices A, B, and D are all explicit in the passage. The passage never states, however, that the symptoms of disease do not emerge until the body has learned how to fight the disease-causing microbe. On the contrary, the passage implies that a person may become quite sick and even die before the body learns to effectively fight the disease.

3. B: In the third paragraph, the word *virulent* means "malicious." The reading comprehension section of the HESI exam will include several questions that require you to define a word as it is used in the passage. Sometimes the word will be one of those used in the vocabulary section of the exam; other times, the word in question will be a slightly difficult word used regularly in academic and professional circles. In some cases, you may already know the basic definition of the word. Nevertheless, you should always go back and look at the way the word is used in the passage. The HESI exam will often include answer choices that are legitimate definitions for the given word, but which do not express how the word is used in the passage. For instance, the word *virulent* could in some circumstances mean contagious or annoying. However, since the passage is not talking about transfer of the disease and is referring to a serious illness, malicious is the more appropriate answer.

4. C: The author's primary purpose in writing this essay is to inform. The reading comprehension section of the HESI exam will include a few questions that ask you to determine the purpose of the author. The answer choices are always the same: The author's purpose is to entertain, to persuade, to inform, or to analyze. When an author is *writing to entertain*, he or she is not including a great deal of factual information; instead, the focus is on vivid language and interesting stories. *Writing to persuade* means "trying to convince the reader of something." When a writer is just trying to provide the reader with information, without any particular bias, he or she is *writing to inform*. Finally, *writing to analyze* means to consider a subject already well known to the reader. For instance, if the above passage took an objective look at the pros and cons of various approaches to fighting disease, we would say that the passage was a piece of analysis. Because the purpose of this passage is to present new information to the reader in an objective manner, however, it is clear that the author's intention is to inform.

5. A: The subject of this passage is foodborne illnesses. Identifying the subject of a passage is similar to identifying the main idea. Do not assume that the first sentence of the passage will declare the subject. Oftentimes, an author will approach his or her subject by first describing some related, familiar subject. In this passage, the author does introduce the subject of the passage in the first sentence. However, it is only by reading the rest of the passage that you can determine the subject. One way to figure out the subject of a passage is to identify the main idea of each paragraph, and then identify the common thread in each.

6. B: This passage never states that cooked food cannot cause illness. Indeed, the first sentence of the third paragraph states that harmful bacteria can be present on cooked food that is left out for two or more hours. This is a direct contradiction of answer choice B. If you can identify an answer choice that is clearly contradicted by the text, you can be sure that it is not one of the ideas advanced by the passage. Sometimes the correct answer to this type of question will be something that is contradicted in the text; on other occasions, the correct answer will be a detail that is not included in the passage at all.

7. C: In the first paragraph, the word *pathogens* means "disease-causing substances." The vocabulary you are asked to identify in the reading comprehension section of the HESI exam will tend to be health related. The exam administrators are especially interested in your knowledge of the terminology used by doctors and nurses. Some of these words, however, are rarely used in normal conversation, so they may be unfamiliar to you. The best way to determine the meaning of an unfamiliar word is to examine how it is used in context. In the last sentence of the first paragraph, it is clear that pathogens are some substances that cause disease. Note that the pathogens are not diseases themselves; we would not say that an uncooked piece of meat "has a disease," but rather that consuming it "can cause a disease." For this reason, answer choice C is better than answer choice A.

8. A: In the second paragraph, the word *sterile* means "free of bacteria." This question provides a good example of why you should always refer to the word as it is used in the text. The word *sterile* is often used to describe "a person who cannot reproduce." If this definition immediately came to mind when you read the question, you might have mistakenly chosen answer D. However, in this passage the author describes raw foods as *not sterile*, meaning that they contain bacteria. For this reason, answer choice A is the correct response.

9. C: The main idea of the passage is that both the esophagus and the stomach are subject to bleeding problems. The structure of this passage is simple: The first paragraph discusses bleeding disorders of the esophagus, and the second paragraph discusses bleeding disorders of the stomach. Remember that statements can be true, and can even be explicitly stated in the passage, and can yet not be the main idea of the passage. The main idea given in answer choice A is perhaps true, but is too general to be classified as the main idea of the passage.

10. B: The passage never states that ulcer disease rarely occurs in the stomach. On the contrary, in the second paragraph the author states that ulcer disease *can* affect the blood vessels in the stomach. The three other answer choices can be found within the passage. The surest way to answer a question like this is to comb through the passage, looking for each detail in turn. This is a time-consuming process, however, so you may want to follow any initial intuition you have. In other words, if you are suspicious of one of the answer choices, see if you can find it in the passage. Often you will find that the detail is expressly contradicted by the author, in which case you can be sure that this is the right answer.

11. A: In the first paragraph, the word *rupture* means "tear." All of the answer choices are action verbs that suggest destruction. In order to determine the precise meaning of rupture, then, you must examine its usage in the passage. The author is describing a condition in which damage to a vein causes internal bleeding. Therefore, it does not make sense to say that the vein has *collapsed* or *imploded*, as neither of these verbs suggests a ripping or opening in the side of the vein. Similarly, the word *detach* suggests an action that seems inappropriate for a vein. It seems quite possible, however, for a vein to *tear*: Answer choice A is correct.

12. D: In the second paragraph, the word *erode* means "wear away." Your approach to this question should be the same as for question 11. Take a look at how the word is used in the passage. The author is describing a condition in which ulcers degrade a vein to the point of bleeding. Obviously, it is not appropriate to say that the ulcer has *avoided*, *divorced*, or *contained* the vein. It *is* sensible, however, to say that the ulcer has *worn away* the vein.

13. A: The primary subject of the passage is a new artificial retina. This question is a little tricky, because the author spends so much time talking about the experience of Kathy Blake. As a reader, however, you have to ask yourself whether Mrs. Blake or the new artificial retina is more essential to the story. Would the author still be interested in the story if a different person had the artificial retina? Probably. Would the author have written about Mrs. Blake if she hadn't gotten the artificial retina? Almost certainly not. Really, the story of Kathy Blake is just a way for the author to make the artificial retina more interesting to the reader. Therefore, the artificial retina is the primary subject of the passage.

14. B: In the second paragraph, the word *progressive* means "gradually increasing." The root of the word is *progress*, which you may know means "advancement toward a goal." With this in mind, you may be reasonably certain that answer choice B is correct. It is never a bad idea to examine the context, however. The author is describing *progressive visual loss*, so you might be tempted to select answer choice C or D, since they both suggest loss or diminution. Remember, however, that the adjective *progressive* is modifying the noun *loss*. Since the *loss* is increasing, the correct answer is B.

15. C: The passage never states that retinitis pigmentosa (RP) is curable. This question may be somewhat confusing, since the passage discusses a new treatment for RP. However, the passage never declares that researchers have come up with a cure for the condition; rather, they have developed a new technology that allows people who suffer from RP to regain some of their vision. This is not the same thing as curing RP. Kathy Blake and others like her still have RP, though they have been assisted by this exciting new technology.

16. D: The author's intention in writing this essay is to inform. You may be tempted to answer that the author's intention is to entertain. Indeed, the author expresses his message through the story of Kathy Blake. This story, however, is not important by itself. It is clearly included as a way of explaining the new camera glasses. If the only thing the reader learned from the passage was the story of Kathy Blake, the author would probably be disappointed. At the same time, the author is not really trying to persuade the reader of anything. There is nothing controversial about these new glasses: Everyone is in favor of them. The mission of the author, then, is simply to inform the reader.

17. A: The main idea of the passage is that Usher syndrome is an inherited condition that affects hearing and vision. Always be aware that some answers may be included in the passage but not the main idea. In this question, answer choices B and D are both true details from the passage, but neither of them would be a good summary of the article. One way to approach this kind of question is to consider what you would be likely to say if someone asked you to describe the article in a single sentence. Often, the sentence you come up with will closely mimic one of the answer choices. If so, you can be sure that answer choice is correct.

18. D: In the first paragraph, the word *symptoms* means "perceptible signs." The word *symptoms* is used frequently in medical contexts, though many people do not entirely understand its meaning.

Symptoms are only those signs of illness that can be observed by someone besides the person with the illness. A stomachache, for instance, is not technically considered a symptom,since it cannot be observed by anyone other than the person who has it. A rash, however, is considered a symptom because other people can see it. The best definition for *symptoms*, then, is perceptible signs; that is, signs that can be perceived.

19. B: The passage does not state that Usher syndrome affects both hearing and smell. On the contrary, the passage only states that Usher syndrome affects hearing and vision. You should not be content merely to note that sentence in the passage and select answer choice B. In order to be sure, you need to quickly scan the passage to determine whether there is any mention of problems with the sense of smell. This is because the mention of impaired hearing and vision does not make it impossible for smell to be damaged as well. It is a good idea to practice scanning short articles for specific words. In this case, you would want to scan the article looking for words like *smell* and *nose*.

20. C: In the second paragraph, the word *juvenile* means "occurring in children." Examine the context in which the word is used. Remember that the context extends beyond just the immediate sentence in which the word is found. It can also include adjacent sentences and paragraphs. In this case, the word juvenile is immediately followed by a further explanation of Usher syndrome as it appears in children. You can be reasonably certain, then, that juvenile Usher syndrome is the condition as it presents in children. Although the word *juvenile* is occasionally used in English to describe immature or annoying behavior, it is clear that the author is not here referring to a *bratty* form of Usher syndrome.

21. B: In the third paragraph, the word *mutated* means "altered." This word comes from the same root as mutant; a *mutant* is an organism in which the chromosomes have been changed somehow. The context in which the word is used makes it clear that the author is referring to a scenario in which one of the parent's chromosomes has been altered. One way to approach this kind of problem is to substitute the answer choice into the passage to see if it still makes sense. Clearly, it would not make sense for a chromosome to be *selected*, since chromosomes are passed on and inherited without conscious choice. Neither does it make sense for a chromosome to be destroyed, because a basic fact of biology is that all living organisms have chromosomes.

22. D: The main idea of the passage is that the immune system protects the body from infection. The author repeatedly alludes to the complexity and mystery of the immune system, so it cannot be true that scientists fully understand this part of the body. It is true that the immune system triggers the production of fluids, but this description misses the point. Similarly, it is true that the body is under constant invasion by malicious microbes; however, the author is much more interested in the body's response to these microbes. For this reason, the best answer choice is D.

23. C: The passage never states that viruses are extremely sophisticated. In fact, the passage explicitly states the opposite. However, in order to know this you need to understand the word *primitive*. The passage says that viruses are too primitive, or early in their development, to be classified as living organisms. A primitive organism is simple and undeveloped—exactly the opposite of sophisticated. If you do not know the word *primitive*, you can still answer the question by finding all three of the answer choices in the passage.

24. D: In the first paragraph, the word *ideal* means "perfect." Do not be confused by the similarity of the word *ideal* to *idea* and mistakenly select answer choice A. Take a look at the context in which the word is used. The author is describing how many millions of microbes can live inside the human body. It would not make sense, then, for the author to be describing the body as a *hostile* environment for microbes. Moreover, whether or not the body is a confined environment would not seem to have much bearing on whether it is good for microbes. Rather, the paragraph suggests that the human body is a perfect environment for microbes.

25. B: The passage never states that the immune system ignores tumors. Indeed, at the beginning of the third paragraph, the author states that scientists remain puzzled by the body's ability to fight tumors. This question is a little tricky, because it is common knowledge that many tumors prove fatal to the human body. However, you should not take this to mean that the body does not at least try to fight tumors. In general, it is best to seek out direct evidence in the text rather than to rely on what you already know. You will have enough time on the HESI exam to fully examine and research each question.

26. A: In the second paragraph, the word *enlist* means "call into service." The use of this word is an example of figurative language, the use of a known image or idea to elucidate an idea that is perhaps unfamiliar to the reader. In this case, the author is describing the efforts of the immune system as if they were a military campaign. The immune system *enlists* other cells, and then directs these *recruits* to areas where they are needed. You are probably familiar with *enlistment* and *recruitment* as they relate to describe military service. The author is trying to draw a parallel between the enlistment of young men and women and the enlistment of immune cells. For this reason, "call into service" is the best definition for *enlist*.

27. C: The author's primary purpose in writing this essay is to inform. As you may have noticed, the essays included in the reading comprehension section of the HESI exam were most often written to inform. This should not be too surprising; after all, the most common intention of any writing on general medical subjects is to provide information rather than to persuade, entertain, or analyze. This does not mean that you can automatically assume that "to inform" will be the answer for every question of this type. However, if you are in doubt, it is probably best to select this answer. In this case, the passage is written in a clear, declarative style with no obvious prejudice on the part of the author. The primary intention of the passage seems to be providing information about the immune system to a general audience.

28. B: The main idea of the passage is that the Food and Drug Administration (FDA) has a special program for regulating dietary supplements. This passage has a straightforward structure: The author introduces his subject in the first paragraph and uses the four succeeding paragraphs to elaborate. All of the other possible answers are true statements from the passage but cannot be considered the main idea. One way to approach questions about the main idea is to take sentences at random from the passage and see which answer choice they could potentially support. The main idea should be strengthened or supported by most of the details from the passage.

29. D: The passage never states that the Food and Drug Administration (FDA) ignores products after they enter the market. In fact, the entire fourth paragraph describes the steps taken by the FDA to regulate products once they are available for purchase. In some cases, questions of this type will contain answer choices that are directly contradictory. Here, for instance, answer choices A and B cannot be true if answer choice D is true. If there are at least two answer choices that contradict another answer choice, it is a safe bet that the contradicted answer choice cannot be correct. If you are at all uncertain about your logic, however, you should refer to the passage.

30. C: In the third paragraph, the phrase *phased in* means "implemented in stages." Do not be tempted by the similarity of this phrase to the word *fazed*, which can mean "confused or stunned." The author is referring to manufacturing standards that have already been implemented for large manufacturers and are in the process of being implemented for small manufacturers. It would make sense, then, for these standards to be implemented in *phases*: that is, to be *phased in*.

31. A: In the fifth paragraph, the word *deceptive* means "misleading." The root of the word *deceptive* is the same as for the words *deceive* and *deception*. Take a look at the context in which the word is used. The author states that the FDA prevents certain kinds of advertising. It would be somewhat redundant for the author to mean that the FDA prevents *illegal* advertising; this goes without saying. At the same time, it is unlikely that the FDA spends its time trying to prevent merely *irritating* advertising; the persistent presence of such advertising makes this answer choice inappropriate. Left with a choice between *malicious* and *misleading* advertising, it makes better sense to choose the latter, since being mean and nasty would be a bad technique for selling a product. It is common, however, for an advertiser to deliberately mislead the consumer.

32. B: The main idea of the passage is that anemia is a potentially dangerous condition characterized by low numbers of RBCs (red blood cells). All of the other answer choices are true (although answer C leaves out RBCs), but only answer choice C expresses an idea that is supported by the others. When you are considering a question of this type, try to imagine the answer choices as they would appear on an outline. If the passage above were placed into outline form, which answer choice would be the most appropriate title? Which answer choices would be more appropriate as supporting details? Try to get in the habit of imagining a loose outline as you are reading the passages on the HESI exam.

33. D: The passage never states that anemia is rarely caused by blood loss. On the contrary, in the first sentence of the fourth paragraph the author lists three causes of anemia, and blood loss is listed first. Sometimes, answer choices for this type of question will refer to details not explicitly mentioned in the passage. For instance, answer choice A is true without ever being stated in precisely those terms. Since the passage mentions several different treatments for anemia, however, you should consider the detail in answer choice A to be in the passage. In other words, it is not enough to scan the passage looking for an exact version of the detail. Sometimes, you will have to use your best judgment.

34. D: In the third paragraph, the word *oxygenated* means "containing high amounts of oxygen." This word is not in common usage, so it is absolutely essential for you to refer to its context in the passage. The author states in the second paragraph that anemia is in part a deficiency of the red blood cells that carry oxygen throughout the body. Then in the first sentence of the third paragraph, the author states that anemic individuals do not get enough oxygenated blood. Given this information, it is clear that *oxygenated* must mean carrying high amounts of oxygen, because it has already been stated that anemia consists of a lack of oxygen-rich blood.

35. A: In the fifth paragraph, the word *severity* means "seriousness." This word shares a root with the word *severe*, but not with the word *sever*. As always, take a look at the word as it is used in the passage. In the final sentence of the passage, the author states that the treatment for anemia will depend on the *cause and severity* of the condition. In the previous paragraph, the author outlined a treatment for anemia and indicated that the proper response to the condition varies. The author even refers to the worst cases of anemia as being *severe*. With this in mind, it makes the most sense to define *severity* as seriousness.

36. C: The main idea of the passage is that a recent study found no link between caffeine consumption and rheumatoid arthritis (RA) among women. As is often the case, the first sentence of the passage contains the main idea. However, do not assume that this will always be the case. Furthermore, do not assume that the first sentence of the passage will only contain the main idea. In this passage, for instance, the author makes an immediate reference to the previous belief in the correlation between caffeine and RA. It would be incorrect, however, to think that this means answer choice A is correct. Regardless of whether or not the main idea is contained in the first sentence of the passage, you will need to read the entire text before you can be sure.

37. A: The passage never states that alcohol consumption is linked with RA. The passage does state that the new study took into account alcohol consumption when evaluating the long-term data. This is a good example of a question that requires you to spend a little bit of time rereading the passage. A quick glance might lead you to believe that the new study had found a link between alcohol and RA. Tricky questions like this make it even more crucial for you to go back and verify each answer choice in the text. Working through this question by using the process of elimination is the best way to ensure the correct response.

38. A: In the second paragraph, the word *symmetrical* means "affecting both sides of the body in corresponding fashion." This is an example of a question that is hard to answer even after reviewing its context in the passage. If you have no idea what *symmetrical* means, it will be hard for you to select an answer: All of them sound plausible. In such a case, the best thing you can do is make an educated guess. One clue is that the author has been describing a condition that affects the hands and the feet. Since people have both right and left hands and feet, it makes sense that inflammation would be described as *symmetrical* if it affects both the right and left hand or foot.

39. B: The author's primary purpose in writing this essay is to inform. You may be tempted to select answer choice D on the grounds that the author is presenting a particular point of view. However, there is no indication that the author is trying to persuade the reader of anything. One clear sign that an essay is written to persuade is a reference to what the reader already thinks. A persuasive essay assumes a particular viewpoint held by the reader and then argues against that viewpoint. In this passage, the author has no allegiance to any idea; he or she is only reporting the results of the newest research.

40. C: The main idea of the passage is that exercise improves bone health. This short passage has a simple structure: The author presents the thesis (main idea) and then spends the rest of the essay supporting it. When a passage is as clearly organized as this one, there should be little mystery about the main idea. If you look at the first sentences of paragraphs two and three, you will see that both contain the words *exercise* and *bones*. This is a good sign that either answer choice A or C is correct. Once you note that weight-bearing exercise is not discussed until the final paragraph, it seems clear that the correct answer must be C.

41. B: In the first paragraph, the word *vital* means "important." On first looking at this word, you might note its similarity to other words having to do with life and liveliness: *vitality*, *revive*, and *vivacious*, to name just a few. This knowledge can help guide your response, though you shouldn't make any assumptions based on it. Otherwise, you might mistakenly select answer choice D. The author states that exercise is *vital* for healthy bones. It would not make sense to say that exercise is *nourishing* for healthy bones, because it would also be so for unhealthy bones. The author is not describing the condition of healthy bones, but rather how bones can be made healthy. For this reason, it makes the most sense to select answer choice B.

42. C: The passage never states that swimming is not good for the bones. This question is a little bit tricky, because the author does state that non-weight-bearing forms of exercise, including swimming, are not *as* good for the bones as weight-bearing exercises. However, just because swimming is not as good for the bones as running does not mean that it is bad for the bones. In fact, swimming works every major muscle system of the body and contributes to overall health, which includes bone health. Be on guard for questions like this that try to fool you into putting words in the author's mouth.

43. A: In the second paragraph, the word *fractures* means "breaks." In the second paragraph, the author declares that exercise reduces the risk of falls and fractures. To begin with, it makes sense to assume that broken bones would be one of the possible results of a fall. We are all aware that older people are more likely to break their bones by falling in the shower or on the stairs. On occasion, authors will use the word *fracture* to describe a damaged relationship, which may tempt you to select *tiffs*. In this case, however, the context makes clear that the author is describing broken bones.

44. B: The main idea of the passage is that the community library offers numerous resources for medical information. While most of the articles used in the reading comprehension section of the HESI exam will be about scientific or health-related concepts directly, some will touch on health and medicine in a more indirect manner. In this article, the author outlines some of the useful sources of medical information that can be obtained at the local library. Answer choices A and C are true, but do not express the general, overarching message of the article. Answer choice D is not true and is directly contradicted by the article itself.

45. D: In the third paragraph, the word *popular* means "for the general public." This word is more often used to describe someone or something that is well known or liked, so you might be tempted to select answer choice C. Take a look at the word as it is used in the context of the third paragraph, however. The author states that the library contains popular magazines and newspapers and then adds that the library also contains medical journals. Popular magazines and newspapers, then, are not the same thing as professional trade journals. Because the latter are known to be complicated and technical (that is, requiring professional expertise), you can guess that *popular* magazines are for a general reading audience.

46. D: The passage does not state that the articles in popular magazines can be hard to understand. If you are working in order, you can use your knowledge of the word *popular* to figure out the answer to this question. Specifically, you will know that the word describes publications that are written for a general, nonexpert audience. With this in mind, it seems unlikely that the articles would also be hard to understand. The other three details are explicit in the passage, so the answer must be D.

47. A: In the fourth paragraph, the word *technical* means "requiring expert knowledge." Again, some of the details gleaned from your work in the preceding questions can help you. The word *technical* is used to describe medical journals. As has already been shown, the author states that medical journals are written for an expert audience and can be difficult for a nonprofessional to understand. If this is the case, you can infer that the word *technical* must mean requiring expert knowledge, answer choice A.

VocabularyandGeneralKnowledgeAnswerKeyandExplanations

1. A: The best definition for the word *prognosis* is "forecast." A prognosis is a probable result or course of a disease. The prognosis usually includes the likelihood of recovery for the patient. A prognosis is distinct from a *diagnosis*, which is just the description of the patient's condition. Likewise, a *description* is not the same thing as a prognosis, because it does not include a suggestion of what will happen in the future. An *outline* is an organized description of a subject, and therefore is not similar to a prognosis. Finally, a *schedule* is a plan for the future, rather than a prediction.

2. D: The name for a substance that stimulates the production of antibodies is an *antigen*. An antigen is any substance perceived by the immune system as dangerous. When the body senses an antigen, it produces an antibody. *Collagen* is one of the components of bone, tendon, and cartilage. It is a spongy protein that can be turned into gelatin by boiling. *Hemoglobin* is the part of red blood cells that carries oxygen. In order for the blood to carry enough oxygen to the cells of the body, there has to be a sufficient amount of hemoglobin. *Lymph* is a near-transparent fluid that performs a number of functions in the body: It removes bacteria from tissues, replaces lymphocytes in the blood, and moves fat away from the small intestine. Lymph contains white blood cells. As you can see, some of the questions in the vocabulary section will require technical knowledge.

3. C: The best definition for the word *abstain* is "to refrain from." Doctors often ask their patients to abstain from certain behaviors that have a negative impact on health. For example, a patient recovering from a viral infection might be asked to abstain from alcohol, so as to prevent weakening of the immune system. To *offend* is "to annoy or irritate." A health-care worker should take care to avoid offending a patient. *Retrain* means "to teach someone how to do a job again." For instance, a nurse might have to be retrained after a long period of not performing a particular task. To *defenestrate* means "to throw out the window." This word is unlikely to be used in a health context.

4. A: The best synonym for *ominous* as it is used in this sentence is "threatening." An ominous symptom, for instance, is one that suggests the presence of serious disease. The word *emboldening* means "making bold." A patient who is regaining strength might be emboldened to try new and more difficult activities. The word *destructive* means "causing damage, chaos, or loss." A destructive condition or behavior has a negative effect on the patient's health. The word *insightful* means "thoughtful or provocative." As a health practitioner, you should try to be insightful so that you can come up with creative solutions to your patients' problems.

5. D: The word *incidence* means "rate of occurrence." A doctor will often refer to the incidence of a particular disease or condition as a measure of its severity or longevity. *Random events* are referred to as "incidents." *Sterility* means "free of living bacteria and microorganisms." It is absolutely necessary for a medical environment to be sterile so that patients will not get infections. *Autonomy* means "self-control and self-determination." A health-care worker should try to promote the autonomy of the patient whenever possible, although autonomy should never be more important than health and well-being.

6. B: *Hydrophilia* means "water loving." One could say that humans have a hydrophilic body, because our bodies crave constant infusions of water. The word *homologous* means "corresponding or having the same relative position or structure." A *dipsomaniac* is a person who cannot resist alcoholic drinks. Dipsomania is a compulsion that must be treated with behavioral therapy or medications such as Antabuse, which causes a violent physical reaction to alcohol. The word *hydrated* means "full of water or sufficiently full of water." Patients need to be hydrated, and medical workers need to be hydrated while they are performing their duties.

7. A: The closest meaning for the word *occluded* as it is used in this sentence is "closed." Occluded means "blocked or obstructed." The word is commonly used to describe arteries that no longer allow the passage of blood. The word *deformed* means "misshapen or out of the normal shape." Any deformed body part is a cause for concern. The word *engorged* means "overfull, especially of blood or food." The organs of the body may become engorged when they are infected or diseased. *Enlarged* means "made larger."

8. D: The best definition for the word *potent* is "powerful." A strong drug may be referred to as potent. The ability of a man to reproduce is sometimes referred to as his potency. The word *frantic* means "frenzied or anxious." A medical worker should never be frantic when dealing with patients and should do his or her best to keep patients from becoming frantic. The word *determined* means "set on a particular path." Whenever possible, a health-care worker should try to ensure that patients are determined to take the necessary steps toward recovery and good health. The word *feverish* can mean either "having a high temperature" or "being worried and anxious." A feverish patient should be comforted and given plenty of fluids.

9. D: The word *precipitous* as it is used this sentence means "steep." Doctors will often refer to a precipitous change in blood pressure. In general, precipitous changes are dangerous to the health. The word *detached* means "unconnected or aloof." A common example is a detached retina, a condition in which part of the eye becomes disconnected, and vision is damaged. The word *sordid* means "dirty" or "vile." The word *encompassed* means "surrounded or entirely contained within." For instance, a doctor might describe a treatment protocol as encompassing all aspects of the patient's life.

10. C: The word *vital* as it is used this sentence means "essential." Medical workers will often refer to a patient's vital signs, meaning blood pressure, heart rate, and temperature. The word *recommended* means "preferred by some authority." The recommended course of treatment is the one outlined and prescribed by a doctor. The word *discouraged* means "disappointed and doubtful of success." Health-care workers should try to prevent patients from becoming discouraged, since this can further diminish quality of life and chances of recovery. The word *sufficient* means "having enough to accomplish the necessary task." As an example, a doctor might inquire to make sure that a patient is receiving sufficient fluids or food.

11. A: The best definition of the word *insidious* is "stealthy." An insidious disease takes root and develops in the body slowly, so that by the time the patient is aware of it, the damage can be severe and even fatal. Cancer is the classic example of insidious disease, because it may take root in the body and develop for a long period without any perceptible signs or symptoms. An insidious disease may be *deadly*, but it is not necessarily so. The words *collapsed* and *new* have no innate relationship to the word *insidious*.

12. B: The word *ingest* means "take into the body." The rate at which a patient ingests food and fluids is important when establishing a treatment protocol. To *congest* is "to fill to excess or to overcrowd." Chest congestion is a common complaint, which may be rooted in serious or minor causes. To *collect* is "to gather together." A health-care worker needs to collect information on patients so as to serve them effectively. To *suppress* means "to hold down or hold back." Patients should be encouraged not to suppress any information during a medical examination; keeping important facts from the doctor or nurse can prevent effective treatment.

13. D: The word *proscribe* means "forbid." A doctor often will proscribe certain foods or behaviors if they would negatively impact patient health. To *anticipate* is "to expect ahead of time." A doctor tries to anticipate how a disease will progress or how a patient will respond to treatment, though it is impossible to do this all the time. To *prevent* is "to keep from happening." Health-care workers try to prevent accidents and mistakes from happening on the job. To *defeat* is "to achieve victory over." The primary goal of treatment is to defeat whatever conditions are adversely affecting the patient's health.

14. C: The word *distended* as it is used in this sentence means "swollen." Doctors will often refer to a distended abdomen, which accompanies gassiness or bloating. The word *concave* means "shaped like the inside of a bowl." Many structures of the human body, for instance the inside of the ear and the arch of the foot, are described as concave. A distended body part may be *sore*, but it is not necessarily so. A distended artery, for instance, may have no accompanying pain. Also, though a distended body part may be *empty*, this is not always the case. In cases of starvation, the stomach may become distended; however, other body parts may become distended from being full to excess.

15. B: The word *overt* as it is used in this sentence means "apparent." Overt signs are those that can be seen by someone other than the person who is experiencing them. A rash is an overt sign; a stomachache is not. The word *concealed* means "hidden." Concealed signs cannot be perceived with the senses; a rise in blood pressure, for instance, is a concealed sign of illness. The word *expert*, used as an adjective, means "knowledgeable about a particular subject." When dealing with an unfamiliar situation, for instance, a doctor might call in an expert practitioner. The word *delectable* means "tasty or delicious."

16. A: The word *supplement* means "something added to resolve a deficiency or obtain completion." A doctor might recommend a particular nutritional supplement to address a patient's needs. A *complement* completes something or makes it perfect. Doctors try to put together complementary treatments that will reinforce and support one another. The word *detriment* means "loss, damage, or injury." A patient should be dissuaded from behaviors that will work to their detriment. The word *acumen* means "expertise" or "special knowledge in some area." A health-care worker will develop acumen based on his or her professional experience.

17. D: The word *paroxysm* means "a violent seizure." A patient who is suffering from paroxysms needs to be stabilized and treated immediately. A *revelation* is "a sudden realization or flash of knowledge." Sometimes, a doctor will puzzle over a case until he or she has a revelation and realizes what needs to be done. A *nutrient* is "something that provides nutrition, or sustenance, to the body." Tests may indicate that a patient needs more of a particular nutrient in order to improve his or her health. A *contraption* is "a mechanical device." Health-care workers must learn how to use all sorts of contraptions in order to perform their duties.

18. B: The word *carnivore* means "meat eating." A patient who is not a carnivore might be in danger of anemia (iron deficiency) or other malnutrition. On the other hand, excessive consumption of red meat can lead to heart disease and obesity. *Hungry* means "feeling hunger." The word *infected* means "contaminated by germs." An infected body part needs to be sterilized and treated immediately. The word *demented* means "crazy or insane," especially when this behavior is the result of the condition known as dementia. A demented individual may not be able to make health-related decisions.

19. C: The word *belligerent* means "pugnacious." *Pugnacious* means "ready to fight." Belligerent patients may be resistant to treatment and disdainful of the doctor's or nurse's authority. The word *retired* means "withdrawn from business." The word *sardonic* means "mocking or sneering." This word is unlikely to come up in a medical context, though a health-care worker should avoid being sardonic. The word *acclimated* means "used to or accustomed to." Often, it takes a while for patients to become acclimated to a course of treatment or to a new lifestyle imposed upon them by diminishing health.

20. A: The word *bilateral* means "on both sides." This word is typically used to describe conditions that afflict both sides of the body. For instance, a patient suffering from bilateral partial paralysis might have numbness in both his right and left arms. The word *insufficient* means "lacking in necessary qualities." A patient might have insufficient blood flow to a certain area, or an insufficient amount of a certain nutrient. A *bicuspid* is anything that ends in two points. Many teeth are referred to as bicuspids because of their shape. The word *congruent* means "agreeing or in complete accord."

21. A: The word *recur* as it is used in this sentence means "occur again." Doctors often refer to the recurrence of a disease or symptom. In some cases, the recurrence of a disease indicates that the treatment used in the past was ineffective. *Recur* has the same root as *occur*, with the prefix *re-*, meaning "back or again." To *survive* means "to remain alive." To *collect* means "to bring together into one place." To *desist* means "to cease or stop doing something." A doctor might advise a patient to desist from a certain behavior in order to improve his or her health.

22. C: The word *labile* means "likely to change." This word is often used as a synonym for unstable. Blood pressure that fluctuates rapidly may be described as labile. The word *venereal* is used to describe conditions that relate to sexual intercourse. Venereal disease, for instance, is acquired during sexual contact. Chlamydia, gonorrhea, and syphilis are all examples of venereal disease. The word *motile* means "moving or capable of moving." A doctor will often refer to a part of the body as motile when its movements have been compromised in the past. An *entrail* is one of the internal parts of an animal or human body. It most often refers to the intestines.

23. B: The best description for the word *flaccid* is "limp." A flaccid part of the body is lacking in muscle tone. The word *defended* means "driven danger away from." The word *slender* means "thin or skinny, but not to the extent of being unhealthy." In general, patients who are slender recover better from injury and illness than patients who are overweight or obese. The word *outdated* describes "something that has become irrelevant with age." As medical technology becomes increasingly sophisticated, much of the equipment that used to be essential has now become outdated.

24. D: The word *androgynous* means "both male and female." Some children are born with androgynous characteristics, and their sexuality may remain ambiguous (hard to determine) for their entire life. *Monozygotic* means "derived from one fertilized egg." Identical twins are often referred to as monozygotic because they emerge from an individual zygote (fertilized egg). The word *exogenous* is used to describe "conditions that originate outside of the body." It is not to be confused with *heterogeneous*, which means "having different parts." *Homologous* means "corresponding or having the same relative position." A dog's body is said to be homologous to a cat's because their legs are in the same place.

25. B: The word *terrestrial* means "earthly." It can also be used to refer to things that are from the land rather than from the water. The word *alien*, when used as an adjective, describes "things that are unfamiliar or from an outside source." *Alien* does not only refer to creatures from outer space. A patient who has come down with a mystery ailment might try to identify some contact with alien substances. The word *foreign* is used to describe "people or things that are from some other area or country." In an area where medical procedures are being performed, foreign objects are usually forbidden. The word *domestic* is used to describe "things that are of the home or household."

26. B: The word *untoward* means "improper or unfortunate." Health-care workers should avoid untoward actions when dealing with their patients. This means acting according to the professional code of ethics. *Allocated* means "reserved for a particular purpose." For example, a patient may be put on a specific exercise regimen. The patient then needs to allocate a certain part of the day for this activity, so that it is sure to be done. *Flaccid* means "limp or lacking in muscle tone." If a patient is experiencing any degree of paralysis, the affected part of the body may be flaccid. *Dilated* means "expanded or made larger." The pupils of the eyes become dilated in the dark so that more light can enter the lens.

27. D: The word *endogenous* as it is used in this sentence means "growing from within." Doctors occasionally refer to endogenous cholesterol, which comes from inside the body rather than from the diet. *Contagious* means "capable of spreading from person to person." A person with a contagious disease needs to be kept away from other people. Often, diseases are only contagious for a limited time. *Continuous* means "proceeding on without stopping." If a patient is suffering from continuous back pain, for instance, he or she is experiencing the pain at all times.

28. B: The word *symptom* means "indication." A symptom is any subjective indication of disease. A symptom can be perceived only by the patient. Lower back pain, for instance, is a symptom, because it cannot be perceived by anyone else. Symptoms are distinct from signs, which are apparent to the patient and other people. Bleeding and high blood pressure are both signs. In medicine, an *indication* is "a sign or symptom that suggests a particular treatment." For example, some rashes are an indication for topical ointment. A *side effect*, on the other hand, is "any effect in addition to the intended effect." The term is often used to describe the unpleasant additional effects of treatment or medication. As an example: Side effects of chemotherapy are nausea and fatigue. A *precondition* is "something that must happen or be true before something else can happen." For example, when a patient has the flu, keeping liquids down is a precondition for trying to eat solid foods.

29. C: The word *invasive* means "intrusive." An invasive disease seeks to penetrate the body and cause damage. Strep throat, a bacterial infection, is an example of an invasive disease. The word *convulsive* means "afflicted by spasms or seizures." A patient who suffers from epilepsy or extreme fever may become convulsive. Convulsive patients need to be stabilized so that they don't hurt themselves. The word *destructive* is used to describe "things that cause damage, injury, or loss." Health-care workers try to steer patients away from destructive behaviors. The word *connective* is used to describe "structures that bring other things into contact." The connective tissues of the body include cartilage, ligaments, and tendons.

30. A: The word *parameter* means "guideline." A doctor will often lay out certain parameters at the beginning of treatment. These are not specific rules, but rather they are the general ideas that will inform the entire course of treatment. Parameters are the boundaries of treatment. A *standard*, on the other hand, is "an established basis of comparison." A *manual* is "a book that explains how to perform a particular task." A *variable* is "something that changes." The amount of food a patient is given might be considered to be a variable, for example.

31. B: The word *void* means "empty." Doctors may refer to a patient's bowels as void when they do not contain any digested food matter. *Holistic* means "concerned with the whole of something rather than with the particular parts." Doctors try to put together a holistic treatment plan so that the patient's general level of health will be improved. *Concrete* is a building material, but the word is also used as an adjective to describe "things that are real, sturdy, and well established." Doctors try to establish concrete standards for measuring a patient's condition, rather than relying on general impressions. *Maladjusted* means "poorly accustomed or acclimated." Although it often takes time for a patient to adjust to a new treatment protocol, some patients will remain maladjusted and require a change in treatment.

32. B: The word *lethargic* as it is used in this sentence means "sluggish." Lethargy is a symptom of many forms of illness. It is also a side effect of chemotherapy. *Nauseous* means "sickened, or suffering from an upset stomach." Nausea is a common side effect of chemotherapy as well; it is just not the one described in this sentence. *Contagious* means "capable of spreading from person to person." Many viral and bacterial infections are contagious. *Elated* means "ecstatic," or "wildly happy." It is usually a good thing when a patient is elated, although manic-depressive patients may alternate between excessive elation and near-suicidal sadness.

33. A: The word *compensatory* means "offsetting." A patient may develop compensatory behaviors to make up for a developing health condition. *Defensive* means "protective" or "intending to repel an attack." Sometimes, patients will feel defensive in the presence of a health professional. *Untoward* means "unfavorable, improper, or unfortunate." Untoward events will inevitably occur during the course of treatment; it is the job of the staff to continue their work regardless. *Confused* means "perplexed or bewildered." Some patients, especially the very young or very old, may become confused during treatment. When confusion is identified, health-care workers should slow down and help the patient feel more comfortable.

34. C: The word *atrophy* means "degeneration or wasting away." Doctors often refer to muscle atrophy, which occurs when a patient is immobile for a long period. Physical therapy and massage are two common ways to prevent muscle atrophy when a patient cannot move because of injury or illness. *Dystrophy* is "weakening, degeneration, or abnormal growth of muscle." You may have heard of muscular dystrophy, a hereditary disease in which the muscles gradually lose their strength. *Entropy* is "the tendency toward chaos and disorder." This term is occasionally used in a medical context to describe a patient's tendency toward decline and decrease in function. It is the job of the health-care worker to fight against entropy. *Apathy* is "a lack of caring." Patients who are suffering from serious injury or illness, especially those who have a poor long-term prognosis, may descend into apathy. A health-care worker should try to use his or her influence to improve mood and combat apathy.

35. D: The best description for the word *discrete* is "separate." Discrete symptoms, for example, are those that do not have any connection to one another, though they spring from the same source. The word *subtle* is used to describe things that are "delicate or mysterious in their meaning or intent." Sometimes, the signs of disease will be subtle. Although today's health-care system has amazing technology for spotting the signs of disease, health-care workers still must be on the lookout for the subtle signs of disease.

36. B: The word *site* as it is used in this sentence means "location." Doctors will often refer to the site of an injection or a planned surgery. A *syringe* is "the device used to inject or withdraw fluid from the body." Medical personnel who specialize in withdrawing blood from patients are called phlebotomists. An *artery* is "a blood vessel that carries blood away from the heart to nourish the rest of the body." Although the site to which the author is referring in this sentence is a *hole*, it will not always be so. For this reason, "hole" cannot be the best definition for *site*.

37. A: The word *exposure* as it is used in this sentence means "laying open." The most common usage of this term is in reference to the sun, although exposure to toxic chemicals is also a major health concern. A doctor will often ask a patient to limit his or her exposure to some environmental element. *Prohibition* is "the act of forbidding." Often, a doctor will place a prohibition on certain behaviors or foods if they are believed to adversely affect health. The words *connection* and *dislike* have no relation to exposure.

38. B: The word *exacerbate* means "aggravate." The first commandment of medical care is "do no harm," which essentially means do nothing to exacerbate the patient's illness or injury. Behaviors or foods that exacerbate the symptoms of illness or injury should be stopped immediately. To *implicate* is "to demonstrate involvement or assign blame." Often, during the examination period, a doctor or nurse will implicate seemingly unrelated behaviors in a patient's condition. Once a behavior has been implicated, the doctor and patient will work together to eliminate its negative effects on health. To *decondition* is "to weaken or diminish the conditioned response to a certain stimulus." Part of working in health care is helping people make positive choices. In part, this is accomplished by deconditioning them to stimuli that provoke a negative response.

39. C: The word *neuron* means "nerve cell." The human body has millions of neurons, with billions of connections between them. A *neutron* is "the part of an atom that has neither positive nor negative charge." Neutrons are located in the nucleus of the atom. The *nucleus* is "the central part of a cell or atom, around which the other parts cluster." The HESI exam requires you to know the names and functions of all the cell parts. *Neutral* means "not taking part in or not taking sides in a dispute." A neutral behavior or medication is one that has neither a positive nor a negative effect on health.

40. B: The word *adverse* means "unfavorable." Unhealthy behaviors have an adverse effect on well-being. *Liberated* means "freed." The general goal of health care is to liberate patients from the negative effects of illness or injury. *Convenient* means "easily accessible and available." When health care is convenient, patients are more likely to acquire it. Health-care workers should strive to make their services convenient for patients whenever possible. *Occluded* means "blocked or closed." Patients with a high level of cholesterol are at risk of developing occluded arteries. Another instance in which the term is used is when a patient is choking: In this case, the patient's airway is said to be occluded.

41. D: The word *holistic* as it is used in this sentence means "concerned with the whole rather than the parts." Doctors try to consider the patient's health from a holistic perspective; that is, they try to improve health in its entirety rather than to eliminate specific symptoms. The word *insensitive* means "not responsive." The word *ignorant* means "lacking knowledge." Health-care workers cannot be ignorant of the latest findings and information in their field. The word *specialized* means "adapted to or trained in a specific discipline or task." Because of the technological complexity of modern medical practice, most careers in health care are specialized.

42. A: The best description for the word *suppress* is "stop." Sometimes, a patient will suppress their symptoms if they are not psychologically ready to face illness. However, the suppression of illness tends to create other problems. Ultimately, it is better not to suppress illness, but to face it directly. To *strain* is "to work hard or overextend." This word is used in a couple of different ways in health care. A patient may be suffering from a specific muscle strain after excessive exercise or hyperextension. Also, a doctor may prohibit a patient from straining in his or her professional life if it is causing fatigue and making the patient vulnerable to disease.

43. D: The word *impending* means "about to happen." A doctor might refer to impending symptoms, which are the symptoms the patient is likely to start experiencing in the near future. *Depending* means "relying on or placing trust in." Because most patients have no medical expertise, they are depending on doctors and nurses to choose the appropriate course of action. *Offending* means "annoying or irritating." *Suspending* means "stopping for an undetermined period." If a treatment is not working, for instance, or if it is causing unforeseen negative side effects, then a doctor may suspend it until more information can be gathered.

44. C: The word *symmetric* as it is used in this sentence means "occurring in corresponding parts at the same time." Some illnesses will cause symmetric rashes, meaning that both the right and left sides of the body are afflicted with similarly shaped inflammation. The word *scabbed* means "covered with wounds." The word *geometric* is used to describe "things that resemble the classic geometric shapes, such as the circle, square, or triangle." On occasion, a doctor may use this word to describe the pattern of a wound or rash.

45. B: The word *patent* means "open." Doctors will describe an artery as patent when it allows a free flow of blood. Similarly, a patent airway allows for unrestricted breathing. *Inverted* means turned upside down or backwards. Sometimes, a patient will be inverted in order to stimulate blood flow to certain parts of the body. A *convent* is "a home for nuns or monks." This word has no relevance to health care, but it is included because the HESI exam will sometimes try to tempt you with answer choices that sound like the right answer. The word *converted* means "changed or altered." A patient may have his or her diet converted in order to meet the needs of a treatment protocol.

46. C: The word *volume* as it is used in this sentence means "quantity." Doctors will refer to an increase in the volume of urine or some other body product as an indication of health. Volume is calculated as length × width × height (or depth); it is a three-dimensional measure. *Length*, on the other hand, is "a two-dimensional measure of distance." *Quality* means "degree of excellence."

Quantity can be measured in any kind of units. *Loudness* might be the right answer if *volume* were being used in a different way, as "the relative power of a sound." In this sentence, however, the word is not being used to describe a sound.

47. D: The word *repugnant* means "offensive, especially to the senses or the morals." For instance, a patient may find a certain kind of medicine repugnant, in which case the doctor must either figure out a way to disguise the taste or consider a different form of treatment. The word *destructive* means "causing damage, injury, or loss." Patients should be steered away from destructive behaviors. *Selective* means "choosy or capable of making a thoughtful choice." In general, it is good to be selective, although a patient who is too selective about his or her diet may develop a nutritional deficiency. *Collective* means "combined or grouped together to form a whole." Health care seeks to treat the collective symptoms of the patient, rather than to focus on specific problems.

48. A: The word *dilate* means "enlarge." Dilation is often expressed as measurement, typically in units of centimeters. For instance, when the body becomes hot, the arteries dilate and blood rushes to the extremities. To *protrude* means "to stick out." Sometimes when a patient breaks a bone severely, part of the bone will protrude from the skin. To *occlude* means "to close up or block." Airways and arteries are the most common parts of the body to become occluded. Either of these occlusions needs to be dealt with immediately before other treatment can be administered.

49. C: The best description for the word *intact* is "unbroken." The word can be used in a number of different contexts. For instance, if a patient presents with severe pain in his or her side, the doctor might worry about the possibility of a ruptured appendix. After an X-ray reveals no damage to the appendix, however, the doctor might say that the organ is intact.

50. C: The word *access* means the ability "to enter, contact, or approach." It is important for patients to have easy access to health-care services. If patients do not have convenient access to services, they will be less likely to take actions to improve health. *Ingress* is "entering or going in." In some cases, a doctor will have to perform tests to determine a disease's path of ingress to the body. *Excess* is "too much or an overabundance of something." In general, excess of any kind is bad for the health. Even excessive exercise can be detrimental to health. During an initial examination, the doctor will try to identify areas in which the patient needs attention. *Success* is "the attainment of goals, whether personal, emotional, professional, physical, or financial." Obviously, the success of the patient is the top priority for all health-care workers.

GrammarAnswerKeyandExplanations

1. C: The word *effected* is not spelled correctly in the context of this sentence. In order to answer this question, you need to know the difference between *affect* and *effect*. The former is a verb and the latter is a noun. In other words, *affect* is something that you do and *effect* is something that is. In this sentence, the speaker is describing something that the prescription medication *did*. Therefore, the appropriate word is a verb. *Effect*, however, is a noun. For this reason, instead of *effected* the author should have used the word *affected*.

2. C: The word *us* makes the sentence grammatically correct. *Us* is the objective case of *we*. In this case, *us* is being used as an indirect object. An indirect object is the noun to which the action of the verb refers. In the sentence *He gave her a sandwich*, the indirect object is *her* (and the direct object is *sandwich*). All of the answer choices for this question are in the first-person plural, with the exception of answer choice D, which is in the third-person plural. The appropriate third-person plural form to complete this sentence is *them*.

3. A: The word *is* makes the sentence grammatically correct. In order to answer this question, you need to determine what the object of the verb will be. One way to do this is to rearrange the question as if it were a declarative sentence: *Picking up the groceries ____ one of the things you are supposed to do.* Expressed like this, it is easy to see that the subject of the sentence is "picking up the groceries." This is a third-person singular subject (that is, it is an "it"), so it receives the third-person present indicative verb form, *is.*

4. D: The word *avoid* makes the sentence grammatically correct. To *avoid* is to keep from doing something. The sentence states that it is impossible to function in the modern world without learning how to use a computer. The word *evade* has a similar meaning to *avoid*, but the verb form used here does not fit into the sentence correctly. The best way to approach this kind of question on the HESI exam is to read the sentence aloud softly, substituting in the various answer choices. If you used this strategy on question 4, you would immediately notice that answer choice B does not correctly complete the sentence.

5. B: The word *hear* is not spelled correctly in the context of this sentence. The speaker has mixed up the homophones *hear* and *here. Homophones* are words that sound the same but are spelled differently and have a different meaning. Homophones are not to be confused with *homonyms*, which are spelled the same but have a different meaning. In question 5, the author is trying to describe the place where the climate is; that is, he or she is describing the climate *here.* Unfortunately, the author uses the word *hear*, which is a verb meaning "to listen."

6. D: The word *our* makes the sentence grammatically correct. *Our* is the possessive case of *we*, In this case, our is being used as an attributive adjective. An adjective is a word that modifies (or describes) a noun. *Our* is called an attributive adjective because it is attributing (assigning) ownership of the screaming to a particular party, *us.* Answer choices A and D are in the first-person plural; answer choices B and C are in the third-person plural. Neither B nor C, however, is in the possessive case. The sentence could be effectively completed with *their*, but this choice is not available.

7. D: The phrase *have to* makes the sentence grammatically correct. The speaker is trying to express that his group was forced to try hard. For this reason, it is essential for the verb *have* to be used. *Have* is an auxiliary verb indicating obligation. It agrees with the first-person plural pronoun *we.* An auxiliary verb accompanies another verb and makes some alterations in mood or tense. In this case, the addition of the verb have indicates that the speaker and others were obliged to try hard. *Can, will*, and *have* are all common examples of auxiliary verbs.

8. D: The word *which* makes the sentence grammatically correct. In this sentence, *which* is used as a relative pronoun. A relative pronoun introduces a relative clause, which is so called because it "relates" to the antecedent. The antecedent is the word that the relative pronoun refers to. In this sentence, the antecedent is "French braid," and the subsequent relative clause gives the reader more information about the French braid. Answer choice C is also a relative pronoun, but it is rarely used after a comma.

9. B: The phrase *toward peace was* makes this sentence grammatically correct. The word *toward* is a preposition that can mean "in the direction of" or "with a view to obtaining." It is in this last sense that the word is being used in this sentence. Peace is an abstract concept, not a physical destination that one could actually reach. For this reason, it does not make sense to select answer choices A or C. Answer choice D has an incorrect verb form; since the subject of the sentence is "working toward peace," the third-person singular verb form is correct.

10. A: The phrase *dog, who had* makes the sentence grammatically correct. To begin with, it is necessary for there to be a comma separating these two clauses, because the second clause is nonrestrictive. A clause is considered nonrestrictive if it could not stand by itself and if the rest of the sentence would still make sense were it removed. If the portion of this sentence after the comma were removed, the sentence would be *Janet called her dog*. Obviously, this is still a coherent sentence. Also, *who* is used here instead of *which* because the antecedent, *dog*, has an identity and personality.

11. B: The word *break* correctly completes this sentence. This question hinges on the different meanings that can be assigned to the word *break*. A *break* can be a brief period of rest from work or some tiring activity, or it can be the act of destroying or disconnecting something. The first usage is as a noun, and the second usage is as a verb. In this sentence, the author is expressing that Dr. Capra needed something, which means you should use the noun form. Also, remember that a *brake* is the mechanism for stopping a vehicle.

12. D: The word *began* properly completes the sentence. The sentence begins with the phrase "the other day," which indicates that the action described took place sometime in the recent past. A past tense verb form is appropriate, then. The verb *begun* is the past participle of *begin*. A past participle describes action that took place before but is now complete. This sentence does not indicate, however, that the action is now complete. For all we know, Stan could still be reviewing his class notes. For this reason, the past tense *began* is the correct answer.

13. C: The word *since* makes the sentence grammatically correct. In this sentence, *since* is being used as a conjunction meaning "because." The word can also be used as an adverb or a preposition indicating an interval from some past time to the present. In this sentence, however, the right answer is indicated by the context. The first part of the sentence states that the current prescription is to be maintained; this suggests that the speaker has a positive attitude toward it. It makes sense, then, that the prescription would have worked well in the past, and that this would be the reason for continuing it.

14. A: The word *rises* makes the sentence grammatically correct. At the heart of this question is the distinction between *rise* and *raise*, which can be summed up in one sentence: To *raise* is to cause to *rise*. This probably requires a little explanation. *Raise* is generally a transitive verb, meaning that it has to be done to something. In other words, it needs an object. One *raises* a window or *raises* a question, but a window or question does not *raise* itself. *Rise*, on the other hand, is typically used as an intransitive verb. This means that it does not take an object. I *rise* from sleep; I do not *rise myself* from sleep. In the sentence for question 14, the blood pressure is doing the action described by the verb, and there is no object. For this reason, *rises* is correct.

15. C: The word *despite* completes the sentence correctly. *Despite* is a preposition meaning "notwithstanding" or "in spite of." A preposition is a word that indicates relationship. *At, by, with,* and *before* are all prepositions. All of the answer choices for question 15 include prepositions. So in order to answer the question, you need to determine which relationship the author is most likely trying to express. The first clause indicates that the two professionals had similar training, and the second clause that indicates they drew different conclusions. It would not make sense for them to draw different conclusions *because of* their similar training; one would expect both professionals to approach a question in the same way. Answer choices B and D create an incoherent statement when they are substituted into the sentence. The answer must therefore be C.

16. D: The word *is* makes the sentence grammatically correct. In order to answer this question correctly, you need to be able to identify the subject. Although it may seem as if the subject is *the two European capitals*, this is actually a clause related to the subject *each*. *Each* is a singular

3 HESI Admission Assessment Practice Tests

pronoun, in which two or more things are being considered individually. In this case, each of these things is an "it," so the appropriate verb form will be the third-person singular present indicative *is*.

17. B: The word *further* is not used correctly in the context of this sentence. Here, the word *farther* would be more appropriate. The distinction between *further* and *farther* is likely to appear in at least one question on the HESI exam. For the purposes of the examination, you just need to know that *farther* can be used to describe physical distance, while *further* cannot. In this sentence, the speaker is describing a distance to be walked, which is a physical distance. For this reason, the word *further* is incorrect.

18. B: The word *sat* is used incorrectly in this sentence. The word *set* would be a good substitution for *sat*. The distinction between *sit* and *set* is likely to appear at least once during the HESI exam. *Sit* is an intransitive verb that does not need an object. One does not *sit* something else, one just *sits*. *Set*, meanwhile, is a transitive verb that requires an object. One *sets* an alarm clock or a table, one does not just *set*. In the sentence on question 18, the little boy is placing something, namely the red block. A transitive verb is required, therefore. For this reason, the past tense of *set* (also *set*) is correct, while the past tense of *sit* (*sat*) is not.

19. B: The phrase *to divulge* makes the sentence grammatically correct. *To divulge* is the infinitive form of a verb meaning to "reveal or disclose information." The verb can stay in the present tense because the speaker is describing what Laura knew at a particular time in the past. In other words, the author has already established the past tense with the word *knew*. It would also be appropriate to fill this blank with the word *divulging*. However, this is not one of the answer choices.

20. C: The word *closely* makes the sentence grammatically correct. Remember that an adjective is a word that describes a noun, while an adverb describes an adjective, a verb, or another adverb. In this sentence, you are looking for the right word to describe how the attendant *looked*. This means that you are looking for an adverb. Most of the time, adverbs end in -*ly*. On question 20, answer choices C and D both have this ending. Answer choice D, however, does not really make sense when substituted into the sentence.

21. B: The word *illusion* is used incorrectly in this sentence. Instead, the author should have used the word *allusion*. An illusion is a false or deceptive image. For example, a magician pulling a rabbit out a hat is a famous illusion. The magician does not actually produce the rabbit out of thin air, but is able to create the image of having done so. An *allusion*, on the other hand, is an indirect reference. If the doctor had said something like, "in light of your past issues," and Henry knew that the doctor meant his depression, then the doctor would have made an allusion.

22. B: The word *should* correctly completes the sentence. All of the answer choices are auxiliary verbs, which are verbs that accompany other verbs and add some element of tone or mood. In order to determine the appropriate auxiliary verb for this sentence, you need to take a close look at the context. The *if* that initiates the sentence suggests that the author is making a conditional statement. In other words, in order to join the club, a condition must be met: Namely, the coach must be contacted by Thursday. For this reason, *should* is the appropriate auxiliary verb. When should is placed before a verb, it adds a note of obligation or recommendation. For instance, saying "you should brush your teeth" is like saying "brushing your teeth is a healthful act that you ought to do."

23. B: The word *set* makes the sentence grammatically correct. This questions centers on the distinction between *set* and *sit*. *Set* is transitive and needs to have an object. This means that it has to be done to something (there are a few exceptions, like *the sun sets*). The past tense and past participle of *set* are both *set*. *Sit*, meanwhile, is intransitive and takes no object. You don't sit something; you just sit. The past tense and past participle of *sit* is *sat*. In this case, the blank must be filled by a transitive verb, because the verb is acting on something else: the law practice. For this reason, *set* is the correct answer.

24. A: The phrase *more efficient* makes the sentence grammatically correct. Here, the author is attempting to describe a comparison between two things: the coal furnace and the woodstove. The comparative form of an adjective usually ends with *-er*: *taller, wiser, cleaner*, for example. In some cases, however, the word *more* is placed in front of the unchanged adjective. As a general rule, multisyllabic words are more likely to use the *more* construction than the *-er* construction. That is the case with *efficient*. Unfortunately, there is no easy rule for memorizing the comparative forms of common English adjectives. Reading is one way to develop a good eye for proper usage.

25. C: The word *has* is used incorrectly in this sentence. The auxiliary verb *have* would be a correct substitution for *has*. *Have* and *has* are auxiliary verbs that, along with *developed*, form a past participle. A past participle is used for action that took place in the past and is now complete. The subject of the sentence is soccer players, which means the verb has to be in the third-person plural. *Has*, however, is the third-person singular. *Have* is in the third-person plural and would therefore be a better choice.

26. A: The word *him* makes the sentence grammatically correct. In this sentence, the blank needs to be filled by a direct object, because you are looking for the person, place, or thing to which the action of the verb is being done. Here, we are looking to identify the person who was asked. For that reason, we need the objective case of *he*, which is *him*. The objective case of *she* is *her*. There will probably be several questions in the grammar section of the HESI exam that require you to differentiate between a pronoun used as a subject and a pronoun used as an object.

27. B: The word *with* makes the sentence grammatically correct. *With* is a preposition that can mean a number of different things. Perhaps the most common meaning of *with* is "in the company of." In this sentence, however, a more accurate meaning is "in regard to." The word *among* is not appropriate here, because progress is not something one could physically be in the middle of. That is, *progress* is not a group of individual things. The word *regards* is not grammatically appropriate for this sentence, although the sentence could be correctly completed with the phrase *with regard to*. Finally, the word *besides* is incorrect because it would not make sense for Felix to not be pleased with his own progress.

28. C: The word *hungrily* makes the sentence grammatically correct. In order to answer this question, you must know the difference between an adjective and an adverb. An adjective modifies a noun. For instance, in the phrase *the delicious meatball*, *delicious* is an adjective. An adverb, on the other hand, modifies an adjective, a verb, or another adverb. In the phrase *walking quickly away*, *quickly* is an adverb. In the sentence for this question, it seems clear that the answer must modify the verb *eyed*. After all, it would not make much sense for the cheesecake to be hungry. This means that an adverb is required. The adverbial form of *hungry* is *hungrily*.

29. C: The word *recipe* is not used correctly in the context of this sentence. The author of this sentence has apparently confused the word *recipe* and *receipt*. A *recipe* is a list of instructions for making something, usually a food or beverage. You might have a recipe for chocolate chip cookies, for instance. A *receipt*, on the other hand, is a printed acknowledgement of having received a certain amount of money and goods. The slip of paper you are handed after paying for something in a store is a receipt. The HESI exam will most likely contain a few questions that require you to identify mixed-up word choices.

30. B: The word *good* properly completes this sentence. This question centers on the distinction between good and well, and, more generally, between adjectives and adverbs. An adjective is used to describe a noun or a pronoun. In the phrase *the red bicycle*, for example, *red* is an adjective describing *bicycle*. An adverb, on the other hand, describes a verb, an adjective, or another adverb. Words that end in *-ly* are usually adverbs, describing the way something is done. As an example, in the phrase *running steadily*, *steadily* is an adverb. To succeed on the HESI exam, you need to know that *good* is an adjective and *well* is an adverb. In question 30, you are looking for a word that describes how Sharon felt, not one that describes her act of feeling. For this reason, you should select the adjective *good*.

31. D: The word *lying* is used incorrectly in this sentence. It would be correct to use the verb *laying* instead. The distinction between *laying* and *lying* is tricky. *Laying* is typically used as a transitive verb, meaning that it is done to something. One lays bricks or lays carpet, for instance. Lie, on the other hand, is an intransitive verb: It is not done to something; it is just done. You *lie* on the floor, for instance. The definition of *lay* is to place; to *lie* is to take ahorizontal position. In this sentence, the subject (Brendan) is laying something (bricks), so it is incorrect to use the verb *lying*.

32. A: The word *who* makes the sentence grammatically correct. In this sentence, *who* is being used as a relative pronoun: that is, a pronoun introducing a clause that describes a noun already mentioned. The noun being referred to, known as the antecedent, is *children*. Because children are people with a personality and identity, the pronoun *who* is used rather than *which*. *Which* is used as a relative pronoun when the antecedent is an inanimate object, such as a box or a house.

33. C: The word *struck* makes the sentence grammatically correct. *Struck* is the past tense and past participle of *strike*, meaning "to hit" or "to beat." *Striked* is not a word. In this case, however, the author is using the common expression "struck a bargain." This expression is frequently used to describe deal making or the end of negotiations. These kinds of conversational phrases may be especially difficult for students whose native language is not English. If you are unfamiliar with expressions in English, you may want to pick up a glossary of slang or colloquial expressions.

34. A: The phrase *him or her* makes the sentence grammatically correct. In this case, we are looking for a word or words that can serve as the object of the preposition *for*. *She* and *he* are nominative forms, meaning that they can only be used as the subject of a sentence or a clause. *Them* can be the object of a preposition, but it is plural and, therefore, cannot correctly refer to the singular subject *a child*. (Incidentally, the use of *they* and *them* to refer to a singular subject is one of the most common grammatical errors, and will almost certainly appear in one or more questions on the HESI exam.) For a similar reason, you cannot use *it* to refer to *a child*. The correct answer, then, is *him or her*.

35. A: The word *swam* makes the sentence grammatically correct. *Swam* is the past tense of the verb *swim*. The context of this sentence makes clear that the action took place in the past; the author uses the past tense verb *was* and describes an action that has already been completed. *Swimmed* is an incorrect verb form. *Swum* is the past participle of *swim*; it would be appropriate if the sentence read *he had swum* or *he has swum*. The absence of these auxiliary verbs means that the simple past tense is appropriate here.

36. C: The phrase *she and I* makes the sentence grammatically correct. The blank needs to be filled by the subject of the sentence. The subject of a sentence or clause is the person, place, or thing that performs the verb. There are a couple of ways to determine that this sentence needs a subject. To begin with, the blank is at the beginning of the sentence, where the subject most often is found. Also, when you read the sentence, you will notice that it is unclear who went to the movies. Because you are looking for the subject, you need the nominative pronouns *she and I*.

37. C: The word *set* makes the sentence grammatically correct. This question requires knowledge of the distinction between *set* and *sit*. *Set* is a transitive verb meaning "to place in a particular position." Transitive verbs have to be done *to* something. *Sit*, meanwhile, is an intransitive verb meaning "to assume a seated posture." In this case, Brian is performing the action of the verb on something in particular: the alarm clock. For this reason, the verb *set* is appropriate.

38. B: The word *shaked* is incorrect in this sentence. In fact, *shaked* is not a word at all. The past tense of *shake* is *shook*. This is similar to the word *take*, which has as its past tense *took* rather than *taked*. There is no real reason for this, making it yet another usage pattern in English that does not conform to any strict rules. After all, the past tense of *wake* is *waked* rather than *wook*. There is no easy way to know all of these rules and exceptions, but a good way to acquire a sense of standard English usage is to become widely read and use a dictionary.

39. B: The word *whichever* makes the sentence grammatically correct. In this sentence, *whichever* is being used as an adjective modifying *way*. The presence of this adjective indicates that Ted was looking in any number of different ways. *Moreover* is an adverb meaning "in addition" or "besides." *Whomever* is the form of whoever used as a direct object, indirect object, or object of a preposition. *Whether* is a conjunction that suggests alternatives or sets of two choices.

40. C: The word *lain* properly completes the sentence. On this question, the presence of the word *had* is the biggest clue to the right answer. *Had* indicates that the verb phrase is being used as a past participle. A past participle is the verb form used to describe action that took place in the past and has been completed. In other words, the treasure started lying there a long time ago, and its position was fully established in the past. Remember that *lain* is the past participle of *lie*, and *laid* is the past participle of *lay*. The verb here is clearly intransitive (that is, it does not act on something else, it just does something), so the correct form is *lain*.

41. B: The word *fewer* makes the sentence grammatically correct. The distinction between fewer and less will most likely appear on your HESI exam. In general, *fewer* is used for things that can be counted and *less* is used for things that cannot be counted. So, for instance, one would say "fewer attendees at this year's conference" and "less confidence in the economy." In this sentence, the adjective is modifying *patients*, who of course can be counted quite easily. So, the correct answer is *fewer*.

42. B: The word *after* makes the sentence grammatically correct. *After* is a conjunction meaning "behind in place or position." A conjunction is a part of speech that connects different words, phrase, and ideas. *And*, *but*, and *because* are all conjunctions. In order to find the appropriate word to complete the sentence in question 42, you need to take a close look at the context. The sentence indicates that Kim realized she had forgotten her list of questions at some time relating to the interview. In other words, it seems clear that the blank must be completed with some word relating to time. Kim either made this realization before, during, or after the interview. Since *after* is one of the answer choices, it must be the correct answer.

43. D: The word *one* is used incorrectly in this sentence. Here, *one* is being used as a pronoun: a stand-in for some other noun. The problem is that it is unclear to what it is referring. The only possible reference for *one* is video store, and it does not make sense to say that "we should rent a video store." Most of the time, we would read this sentence and just assume that the author meant that we should rent a video. However, on the HESI exam, you must be alert for unclear wording.

44. A: The word *who* makes this sentence correct. *Who* is an interrogative pronoun that can be either singular or plural. A pronoun is a word that stands in for another noun. In this case, the pronoun is used so that the author can inquire about the noun to which the pronoun is referring.

Once the question is answered, the names of the best eye doctors could be substituted for *who* to make a complete sentence. In any case, *who* is appropriate because the pronoun is referring to people who have both personality and identity; if they were objects, it would be appropriate to use *which* or *what*. *Whom* is a pronoun in the objective cases and is therefore not appropriate for this sentence.

45. B: The word *spent* makes this sentence grammatically correct. The sentence is clearly describing action that took place in the past, because the introductory clause begins with the word *while*. It cannot be determined whether this action is ongoing or has been completed. The past tense of the verb *spend* is *spent*. Unfortunately, there is no rule to guide this past tense; as a matter of fact, the past tense of the verb *mend* is *mended*, which might lead you to believe that *spended* is correct. Reading a variety of materials is the best way to develop an ear for proper usage.

46. A: The word *amount* correctly completes this sentence. This question centers on the distinction between *amount* and *number*. An *amount* is a quantity that cannot be counted, while a *number* is a quantity that can be counted. There is no way to count pain, so *amount* is a better word choice than *number*. *Frequency* is rate of occurrence, or how often something happens. If a doctor asks how often a patient gets a migraine, for instance, she is asking about the *frequency* of the headaches. *Amplitude* is the specific breadth or width. Amplitude is mainly used to describe waves; the difference in height between the top of a wave (crest) and the bottom (trough) is the amplitude.

47. C: The word *their* is used incorrectly in this sentence. The problem is that *whoever* as it is used here is a singular subject, while *their* is a plural possessive pronoun. *Whoever* can be either singular or plural, depending on how it is used. In this case, however, because the author is describing a letter writer who forgot to sign the letter, it seems clear that *whoever* is meant as a singular. For this reason, the author should use *his or her* instead of *their*.

48. C: The word *too* makes the sentence grammatically correct. Clearly, the author is trying to express that the child's fever was excessively high. Of the four answer choices, three convey this idea. Only answer choice A (the preposition *to*) can be immediately eliminated. The best way to find the final answer is to substitute each of the answer choices into the sentence and read the result. Answer choice B requires the addition of the word *too* to make any sense. Answer choice C, then, must be the correct answer.

49. B: The word *presents* makes the sentence grammatically correct. The author is referring to the symptoms that will be displayed when a patient has a particular condition: that is, the presentation of the condition. Because the subject of the sentence (*condition*) is singular, it is proper to use the verb form ending in an *s*. For this reason, you should select answer choice B rather than answer choice C. *Presence* is the quality of being there. When a teacher is calling roll and a student responds to his name by saying "present," he is using a form of this word to indicate that he is there. Of course, *present* can also mean a gift. *Prescience*, on the other hand, is foreknowledge, or knowledge ahead of time. You can exercise prescience by learning the content of the HESI exam and practicing with this study guide.

50. B: The preposition *among* is not used correctly in the context of the sentence. In this case, the word *between* would be more appropriate. *Among* and *between* both mean "in the midst of some other things." However, *between* is used when there are only two other things, and *among* is used when there are more than two. For example, it would be correct to say "between first and second base" or "among several friends." In this sentence, the preposition *among* is inappropriate for describing placement amid "two treatment protocols."

MathematicsAnswerKeyandExplanations

1. A: The answer is 2512. To solve this problem, you must know how to add numbers with multiple digits. It may be easier for you to complete this problem if you align the numbers vertically. The crucial thing when setting up the vertical problem is to make sure that the place values are lined up correctly. In this problem, the larger number (2038) should be placed on top, such that the 8 is over the 4, the 3 is over the 7, and so on. Then add the place value farthest to the right. In this case, the 4 and the 8 that we find in the ones place have a sum of 12; the 2 is placed in the final sum, and the 1 is carried over to the next place value to the left, the tens. The tens place is the next to be added: 3 plus 7 equal 10, with the addition of the carried 1 making 11. Again, the first 1 is carried over to the next place value. The problem proceeds on in this vein.

2. C: The answer is 34,481. This problem requires you to understand addition of multiple-digit numbers. As in the first problem, the most important step is properly aligning the two addends in vertical formation, such that the final 8 in 32,788 is above the final 3 in 1693. Again, as in the first problem, you will be required to carry numbers over. It is a good idea to practice these addition problems and pay special attention to carrying over, since errors in this area can produce answers that look correct. The administrators of the HESI exam will sometimes try to take advantage of these common errors by making a couple of the wrong answers the results one would get by failing to carry over a digit.

3. B: The answer is 1854. To solve this problem, you must know how to subtract one multiple-digit number from another. As with the above addition problems, the most important step in this kind of problem is to set up the proper vertical alignment. In subtraction problems, the larger number must always be on top, and there can be only two terms in all (an addition problem can have an infinite number of terms). In this problem, the ones places should be aligned such that the 3 in 3703 is above the 9 in 1849. This problem also requires you to understand what to do when you have a larger value on the bottom of a subtraction problem. In this case, the 3 on the top of the ones place is smaller than the 9 beneath it, so it must borrow 1 from the number to its left. Unfortunately, there is a 0 to the left of the three, so we must extract a 1 from the next place over again. The 7 in 3703 becomes a 6, the 0 becomes a 10 only to have 1 taken away, leaving it as a 9. The 3 in the ones place becomes 13, from which we can now subtract the 9.

4. A: The answer is 1816. This problem requires you to understand subtraction with multiple-digit numbers. As in problem 3, the most important step is to align the problem vertically such that the 0 in 4790 is above the 4 in 2974. Again as in problem 3, you will have to borrow from the place value to the left when the number on the bottom is bigger than the number on top. Be sure to practice this kind of problem with special attention to borrowing from adjacent place values. The HESI exam will often include a few wrong answers that you could mistakenly derive by simply forgetting how to borrow.

5. C: The answer is 169,002. To solve this problem, you must know how to multiply numbers with several digits. These problems often intimidate students because they produce such large numbers, but they are actually quite simple. As with the above addition and subtraction problems, the crucial first step is to align the terms vertically such that the 8 in 738 is above the 9 in 229. In multiplication, it is a good idea to put the larger number on top, although it is only essential to do so when one of the terms has more place values than the other. In a multiple-digit multiplication problem, every digit gets multiplied by every other digit: First the 9 in 229 is multiplied by the three digits in 738, moving from right to left. Only the digit in the ones place is brought down; the digit in the tens place is placed above the digit to the immediate left and added to the product of the next multiplication. In this problem, then, the 9 and 8 produce 72: The 2 is placed below, and the 7 is placed above the 3 in 738. Then the 9 and the 3 are multiplied and produce 27, to which the 7 is added, making 24. The 4 comes down, the 2 goes above the first 2 in 229, and the process continues. The product of 9 multiplied by 738 is placed below and is added to the products of 2 and 738 and 2 and 738, respectively. For each successive product, the first digit goes one place value to the left. So, in other words, 0 is placed under the 2. These three products are added together to calculate the final product of 738 and 229.

6. D: The answer is 287,648. This problem requires you to understand multiplication of numbers with several digits. The difficulties you may face with this problem are identical to those of problem 5. Be sure set up your vertical alignment properly, such that the 8 in 808 is above the 6 in 356. Multiply the 6 in 356 by 8, 0, and 8, proceeding from right to left. Then multiply the 5 in 356 by 8, 0, and 8; finally, multiply the 3 in 356 by 8. For each successive product, add one zero at the extreme right of the product. Add the three products together to find your final answer.

7. B: The answer is 62. To solve this problem, you must know how to divide a multiple-digit number by a single-digit number. To begin with, set up the problem as $7\overline{)435}$. Then determine the number of times that 7 will go into 43 (one way to do this is to multiply 7 by various numbers until you find a product that is either 43 exactly or no more than 6 fewer than 43). In this case, you will find that 7 goes into 43 six times. Place the 6 above the 3 in 435 and multiply the 6 by 7. The product, 42, should be subtracted from 43, leaving a difference of 1. Since 7 cannot go into 1, bring down the 5 to create 15. The 7 will go into 15 twice, so place a 2 to the right of the 6 on top of the problem. At this point, you should recognize that only answer choice B can be correct. If you proceed further, however, you will find that 435 must become 435.0 so that the 0 can be brought down to make a large enough number to be divided by 7. Once a decimal point is introduced to the dividend, a decimal point must be placed directly above it in the quotient. If you continue working this problem, you will end up with an answer of 62.14 … Note that the instructions tell you only to round to the nearest whole number. Once you have solved to the tenths place, there is no need to continue.

8. C: The answer is 396. To solve this problem, you must understand division involving multiple-digit numbers. To begin with, set up the problem as $12\overline{)4,748}$. Then solve the problem according to the procedure you followed in problem 7. Since you are asked to round to the nearest whole number, you must solve this problem to the tenths place. If your calculations are correct, you will have a 6 in the tenths place, meaning that the answer should be rounded up from 395 to 396.

9. A: The answer is 14.989. To solve this problem, you must know how to add a series of numbers when some of the numbers include decimals. As with addition problems 1 and 2, the most important first step is to set up the proper vertical alignment. This step is even more important when working with decimals. Be sure that all of the decimal points are in alignment; in other words, the 7 in 3.7 should be above the 2 in 7.289. Since the final term, 4, is a whole number, we assume a 0 in the tenths place. Similarly, you may assume zeros in the hundredths and thousandths places, if you prefer to have a digit in every relevant place. Then beginning at the rightmost place value (in this case, the thousandths), add the terms together as you would with whole numbers. The decimal point of the sum should be aligned with the decimal points of the terms.

10. A: The answer is 21.114. This problem requires you to understand addition involving a series of numbers, some of which include decimals. This problem is solved in the same manner as problem 9. Be sure to align the terms correctly, such that the 9 in 4.934 is above the 1 in 7.1 and the 0 in 9.08. Assume zeros for the hundredths and thousandths place of 7.1 and for the thousandths place of 9.08. The usual rules for carrying in addition still apply when working with decimals.

11. B: The answer is 23.46. To solve this problem, you must know how to subtract a number with a decimal from a whole number. At first glance, this problem seems complex, but it is actually quite simple once you set it up in a vertical form. Remember that the decimal point must remain aligned and that a decimal point can be assumed after the 7 in 27. In order to solve this problem, you should assume zeros for the tenths and hundredths places of 27. The problem is solved as 27.00 – 3.54. Obviously, in order to solve this problem you will have to borrow from the 7 in 27.00. The normal rules for borrowing in subtraction still apply when working with decimals. Be sure to keep the decimal point of the difference aligned with the decimal points of the terms.

12. D: The answer is 19.19. This problem requires you to understand subtraction of a whole number from a number with a decimal. This problem is somewhat similar to problem 11, although here the decimal is on the top in your vertical alignment. Assume zeros for the tenths and hundredths place of the bottom term, creating the problem 28.19 – 9.00. Be sure to keep your decimal point in the same position in the difference as in the terms. HESI exam administrators often try to fool test-takers by including some possible answers that have the correct digits, but in which the decimal point is misplaced.

13. B: The answer is $31.90. To solve this problem, you must know how to solve word problems involving decimal subtraction. In this scenario, Karen starts out with a certain amount of money and spends some of it on groceries. To calculate how much money she has left, simply subtract the money spent from the original figure: 40 – 1.85 – 3.20 – 3.05. There is no reason to include the dollar sign in your calculations, so long as you remember that it exists. You cannot subtract the costs of these items at the same time, so you must either subtract them one by one or add them up and subtract the sum from 40. Either way will generate the right answer.

14. C: The answer is 24.5. This problem requires you to understand multiplication including numbers with decimals. In some ways, multiplying decimals is easier than adding or subtracting them. This is because the decimal points can be ignored until the very end of the process. Simply set this problem up such that the longer term, 277.9, is on top (this term is considered longer because the initial 0 in 0.088 performs no function). Then multiply according to the usual system: Multiply the rightmost 8 by 9, 7, 7, and 2, and then do the same for the next 8. Add the two products together. Finally, count up the number of decimal places to the right of the decimal point in both terms. In this problem, there are four: 0.<u>088</u> and 277.<u>9</u>. This means that there should be four places to the right of the decimal point in the product. Once the product is found, you must round it to the tenths place. This is done by assessing the digit in the place to the right of the tenths place (that is, the hundredths place). If that digit is lower than 5, round down; if it is 5 or greater, round up. In this case, there is a 5 in the hundredths place, so the 4 in the tenths place becomes a 5.

15. A: The answer is 46.67. To solve this problem, you must know how to divide a whole number by a decimal. To begin with, set the problem up in the form $0.6\overline{)28}$. You cannot perform division when the divisor is less than one, however, so shift the decimal point one place to the right. For every action in the divisor, an identical action must be taken in the dividend: Shift the decimal point (which can be assumed after the 8 in 28) in the dividend as well. The problem is now $6\overline{)280}$. This problem can now be solved just like problems 7 and 8. Remember to round your answer to the hundredths place for this problem (this means you will need to solve to the thousandths place). With a knowledge of place value, you can immediately eliminate answer choices B and D, since they are solved to the nearest thousandth and tenth place, respectively.

16. D: The answer is 400 miles. This problem requires you to understand word problems involving mileage rates and multiplication. The problem states that the car gets an average 25 miles per gallon; in other words, every gallon of fuel powers the car for approximately 25 miles. If the car holds 16 gallons of gas, then, and each of these gallons provides 25 miles of travel, you can set up the following equation: 25 miles/gallon × 16 gallons = 400 miles. Since the first term has gallons in the denominator and the second term has gallons in what would be the numerator (if it were expressed as 16 gallons/1), these units cancel each other out and leave only miles.

17. C: The answer is $\frac{5}{8}$. To solve this problem, you must know how to add fractions with like denominators. This kind of operation is actually quite simple. The denominator of the sum remains the same; the calculation is performed by adding the numerators. On problems like this, HESI exam administrators will probably try to fool you by including one possible answer in which the denominators have been added; in this problem, for instance, you would end up with answer choice D if you added both numerator and denominator. Do not assume that you have answered the question correctly because your calculations match one of the answer choices. Always check your work.

18. A: The answer is $\frac{20}{21}$. This problem requires you to understand addition of fractions with unlike denominators. The denominator is the bottom term in a fraction; the top term is called the numerator. In order to perform addition with a fraction, all of the terms must have the same denominator. In order to derive the lowest common denominator in this problem, you must list the multiples for 3 and 7 until you find one that both have in common. In increasing order, multiples of 3 are 3, 6, 9, 12, 15, 18, and 21; multiples of 7 are 7, 14, and 21. The lowest common multiple is 21. This is also the lowest common denominator for the two fractions. To convert each term into a fraction with this common denominator, you must multiply both numerator and denominator by the same number. To make the denominator of $\frac{2}{3}$ into 21, you must multiply by 7; therefore, you must also multiply the numerator, 2, by 7. The new fraction is $\frac{14}{21}$. For the second term, you must multiply numerator and denominator by 3: $\frac{2}{7} \times \frac{3}{3} = \frac{6}{21}$. The new addition problem is $\frac{14}{21} + \frac{6}{21}$. Remember that when adding fractions, only the numerators are combined.

19. D: The answer is $2\frac{5}{6}$. To solve this problem, you must know how to add mixed numbers and improper fractions. To begin with, convert the mixed number (a mixed number includes a whole number and a fraction) into an improper fraction (a fraction in which the numerator is larger than the denominator). This is done by multiplying the whole number by the denominator and adding the product to the numerator: 1 × 2 + 1 = 3. The problem is now $\frac{3}{2} + \frac{12}{9}$. Then find the lowest common denominator by listing some multiples of 2 and 9. The lowest common multiple is 18, so you must convert both terms: $\frac{3}{2} \times \frac{9}{9} = \frac{27}{18}$, and $\frac{12}{9} \times \frac{2}{2} = \frac{24}{18}$. The problem is now $\frac{27}{18} + \frac{24}{18} = \frac{51}{18}$. This fraction is converted into a mixed number by dividing the numerator by the denominator: $\frac{51}{18} = 2\frac{15}{18}$, which can be simplified to $2\frac{5}{6}$ by dividing both numerator and denominator by 3.

20. D: The answer is $13\frac{11}{12}$. This problem requires you to understand addition involving mixed numbers. The calculation required by this problem is straightforward: In order to derive the number of hours worked by Aaron, add up the three mixed numbers. To make this possible, you will need to find the lowest common multiple of 2, 4, and 3, so that you can establish a common denominator. The lowest common denominator for this problem is 12. You can either add up the whole numbers separately from the fractions or convert the mixed numbers into improper fractions and add them in that form. Either way will yield the correct answer.

21. B: The answer is $\frac{1}{2}$. To solve this problem, you must understand subtraction involving fractions with like denominators. As with addition involving fractions with like denominators, you should only subtract the numerators. So, this problem is solved $\frac{23}{24} - \frac{11}{24} = \frac{12}{24}$. This answer can be simplified by dividing by the greatest common factor (a factor is any number that can be divided into the given number equally). The factors of 12 are 1, 2, 3, 4, 6, and 12. The factors of 24 are 1, 2, 3, 4, 6, 8, 12, and 24. The greatest common factor of 12 and 24, then, is 12. Divide both numerator and denominator by 12 to derive the answer in simplest form: $(\frac{12}{12})/(\frac{24}{12}) = \frac{1}{2}$.

22. C: The answer is $1\frac{5}{14}$. This problem requires you to understand subtraction with mixed numbers. In order to perform this problem, you must convert these mixed numbers into improper fractions with the same denominator. Remember that mixed numbers are converted into improper fractions by multiplying the denominator by the whole number and adding the product to the numerator: $3\frac{4}{7}$ becomes $\frac{25}{7}$, and $2\frac{3}{14}$ becomes $\frac{31}{14}$. Next, find the lowest common denominator by listing multiples of 7 and 14. Since 14 is a multiple of 7, you only have to alter the first term. Multiply both numerator and denominator by 2: $\frac{25}{7} \times \frac{2}{2} = \frac{50}{14}$. The problem is now $\frac{50}{14} - \frac{31}{14} = \frac{19}{14}$. Convert this improper fraction into a mixed number by dividing the numerator by the denominator: $\frac{19}{14} = 1\frac{5}{14}$. The mixed number cannot be simplified further.

23. C: The answer is $\frac{1}{2}$. To solve this problem, you must know how to solve word problems requiring fraction addition and subtraction. You are given the proportions of Dean's socks that are white and black. The best approach to this problem is adding together the two known quantities and subtracting the sum from 1. First you need to find a common denominator for $\frac{1}{3}$ and $\frac{1}{6}$. The lowest common multiple of these two numbers is 6, so convert $\frac{1}{3}$ by multiplying the numerator and denominator by 2. The new equation will be $\frac{2}{6} + \frac{1}{6} = \frac{3}{6}$. This sum is equivalent to $\frac{1}{2}$, meaning that half of Dean's socks are either white or black. The other half, then, are brown. If you need to perform the calculation, however, it will look like this:

$$\frac{2}{2} - \frac{1}{2} = \frac{1}{2}.$$

24. A: The answer is $11\frac{2}{3}$. This problem requires you to understand word problems involving the addition and multiplication of mixed numbers and improper fractions. To begin with, convert the three mixed numbers to improper fractions by multiplying the whole number by the denominator and adding the product to the numerator. The resulting fractions will be $\frac{3}{2}$ (sugar), $\frac{11}{3}$ (flour), and $\frac{2}{3}$ (milk). Then find the lowest common multiple of 2 and 3 which is 6 and convert the three fractions so that they have this denominator: $\frac{9}{6}$ (sugar), $\frac{22}{6}$ (flour), and $\frac{4}{6}$ (milk). Add these fractions together and multiply the sum by two to double the recipe: $\frac{9}{6} + \frac{22}{6} + \frac{4}{6} = \frac{35}{6} \times 2 = \frac{70}{6}$ Finally, convert this improper fraction to a simple mixed number by dividing numerator by denominator and simplifying the leftover fraction: $\frac{70}{6} = 11\frac{4}{6} = 11\frac{2}{3}$.

25. D: The answer is $1\frac{5}{21}$. To solve this problem, you must know how to multiply mixed numbers and fractions. Unlike fraction addition and subtraction, fraction multiplication does not require a common denominator. However, it is necessary to convert mixed numbers into improper fractions. This is done by multiplying the whole number by the denominator and adding the product to the numerator: in this case, 4 × 3 + 1 = 13. So the problem is now $\frac{13}{3} \times \frac{2}{7}$. Fraction multiplication is performed by multiplying numerator by numerator and denominator by denominator: (13 × 2)/(3 × 7) = $\frac{26}{21}$. This improper fraction can be converted into a mixed number by dividing numerator by denominator, which gives $1\frac{5}{21}$. Note that since 26 and 21 have no common factors other than 1, the improper fraction cannot be simplified.

26. D: The answer is $\frac{7}{9}$. This problem requires you to understand multiplication of mixed numbers and fractions. The process is the same as for the previous problem: Convert $2\frac{3}{9}$ into the mixed number $\frac{21}{9}$ (if you like, you can simplify this fraction by dividing top and bottom by 3). Then multiply numerator by numerator and denominator by denominator. If you did not simplify the first fraction, you will have a product of $\frac{21}{27}$. This fraction can be simplified by dividing the numerator and denominator by 3: (21/3)/(27/3) = 7/9.

27. D: The answer is $3\frac{1}{8}$. To solve this problem, you must know how to divide fractions. The process of dividing fractions is similar to that of multiplying fractions, except that the second term must be inverted. Once this is done, the numerator is multiplied by the numerator, and the denominator is multiplied by the denominator. The inversion of a number is also known as the reciprocal. So, in this problem, solve by multiplying $\frac{5}{8}$ by the reciprocal of $\frac{1}{5}$, which is $\frac{5}{1}$ (finding the reciprocal of a fraction simply means switching the numerator with the denominator). The problem is solved as $(5 \times 5)/(8 \times 1) = \frac{25}{8}$. Convert this improper fraction into a mixed number according to the usual procedure.

28. D: The answer is $1\frac{5}{7}$. This problem requires you to understand how to divide fractions. The procedure is the same as for the previous problem: Invert the second term and change the problem to one of multiplication: $2/7 \times 6/1 = \frac{12}{7}$. Convert this improper fraction into a mixed number according to the usual procedure. The fraction cannot be simplified because 12 and 7 do not share any factors other than 1.

29. B: The answer is 78. To solve this problem, you must know how to convert a fraction into a ratio. In this problem, you are being asked to convert the fraction into a value on a scale from 1 to 100, which is basically like being asked to convert it into a percentage. To do so, divide the numerator by the denominator. The answer will be a repeating seven: $0.7\overline{777}$. Calculate to the thousandth place in order to determine the value. Because the digit in the thousandths place is a 7, you will round up the digit to the left to establish the final answer, 78.

30. A: The answer is 0.88. This problem requires you to understand the conversion of fractions to decimals. The process is fairly simple: Divide the numerator by the denominator. In order to make this possible, you will have to write 7 as 7.0. The resulting quotient will be 0.875. Remember that the instructions require you to round to the nearest hundredths place. The digit in the thousandths place will be 5, meaning that you need to round up. The final answer is 0.88.

31. B: The answer is 4.43. To solve this problem, you must know how to convert mixed numbers into decimals. Perhaps the easiest way to perform this operation is to convert the mixed number into an improper fraction and then divide the numerator by the denominator. Convert the mixed number into an improper fraction by multiplying the whole number by the denominator and adding the product to the numerator: $4 \times 7 + 3 = 31$, so the improper fraction is $\frac{31}{7}$. Next divide 31 by 7, according to the same procedure used in problems 7 and 8. Remember that when you have to add 0 to 31 in order to continue your calculations, you must put a decimal point directly above in the quotient. Also, since the problem asks you to round to the hundredths place, you must solve the problem to the nearest thousandth.

32. C: The answer is $3\frac{39}{50}$. This problem requires you to understand the conversion of decimals into mixed numbers. 3.78 has value into the hundredths place, so your fraction will have a denominator of 100. There are three whole units and seventy-eight hundredths, a mixed number that can be written as $3\dfrac{78}{100}$. Next, you must simplify this fraction. The only common factor of 78 and 100 is 2; divide both numerator and denominator by 2 to derive the answer, $3\dfrac{39}{50}$. This fraction cannot be simplified any further.

33. C: The answer is $\dfrac{7}{100}$. To solve this problem, you must know how to convert decimals into fractions. Remember that all of the numbers to the right of a decimal point represent values less than one. So, a decimal number such as this will not include any whole numbers when it is converted into a fraction. The 7 is in the hundredths place, so the number is properly expressed as $\dfrac{7}{100}$. The fraction cannot be simplified because 7 and 100 do not share any factors besides one.

34. D: The answer is $2\dfrac{4}{5}$. This problem requires you to understand how to convert a decimal into a fraction or, in this case, a mixed number. Because there are values to the left of the decimal point, you can tell that this number will be equivalent to a mixed number. Indeed, the number 2.80 is equivalent to $2\dfrac{80}{100}$. Next, list the factors of 80 (1, 2, 4, 5, 8, 10, 16, 20, 40, 80) and 100 (1, 2, 4, 5, 10, 20, 25, 50, 100). The greatest common factor is 20, so divide both numerator and denominator by 20 to derive the simplest form of the fraction, $2\dfrac{4}{5}$.

35. B: The answer is 4:7. To solve this problem, you must know how to convert fractions into ratios. A ratio expresses the relationship between two numbers. For instance, the ratio 2:3 suggests that for every 2 of one thing, there will be 3 of the other. If we applied this ratio to the length and width of a rectangle, for instance, we would be saying that for every 2 units of length, the rectangle must have 3 units of width. A fraction is just one way to express a ratio: The fraction $\dfrac{8}{14}$ is equivalent to the ratio 8:14. To simplify the ratio, divide both sides by the greatest common factor, 2. The simplest form of this ratio is 4:7.

36. B: The answer is 9. This problem requires you to understand how to approach word problems involving fractions and ratios. You are given the total number of students in the class and the fraction of students who are boys: With this information, you can determine the number of boys by multiplying $\dfrac{2}{3}$ by 27. You will find that there are 18 boys in the class. You can then find the number of girls by subtracting the number of boys from the total number of students: 27 − 18 = 9. There are nine girls in the class.

37. A: The answer is 16. To solve this problem, you must understand proportions. A proportion is a comparison between two or more equivalent ratios. A simple proportion is 1:2 :: 2:4, which can be expressed in words as "1 is to 2 as 2 is to 4." Just as 2 is twice 1, 4 is twice 2. Problem 37 asks you to identify a missing term in a proportion. One way to do this is to set up the problem as a set of equivalent fractions and solve for the variable: $\dfrac{3}{2}=\dfrac{24}{x}$. To solve this equation, cross-multiply. You will end up with $3x = 48$. To find the value of x, divide both sides by 3.

38. C: The answer is 24. This problem requires you to understand proportions. You can use the same procedure to solve this problem as you used to solve problem 37. Set up the proportion in the same way as a pair of equivalent fractions: $\frac{7}{42} = \frac{4}{x}$. Then solve for x. To do this, you must cross-multiply (producing $7x = 168$), and then divide both sides by 7. Your calculations should determine that $x = 24$.

39. B: The answer is 64%. To solve this problem, you must know how to convert a decimal into a percent. A percentage is a number expressed in terms of hundredths. When we say, for instance, that a candidate received 55% of the vote, we mean that she received 55 out of every 100 votes cast. When we say that the sales tax is 6%, we mean that for every 100 cents in the price another 6 cents are added to the final cost. To convert a decimal into a percentage, multiply it by 100 or just shift the decimal point two places to the right. In this case, by moving the decimal point two places to the right you can derive the correct answer, 64%.

40. A: The answer is 0.0026%. This problem requires you to understand the conversion of decimals into percentages. Remember that percent is equivalent to quantity out of a hundred; 75%, for instance, is 75 out of 100. To convert a decimal into a percentage, then, multiply the given decimal by 100. A simple way to perform this calculation is to shift the decimal point two places to the right. So for this problem, 0.000026 is equivalent to 0.0026%.

41. D: The answer is 0.38. To solve this problem, you must know how to convert percentages into decimals. This is done by shifting the decimal point two places to the right. This operation is the same as dividing the percentage by 100. In this problem, assume that the decimal is after the eight in 38%. The equivalent decimal, then, is 0.38.

42. C: The answer is 0.176. This problem requires you to understand the conversion of percentages into decimals. A percentage is an amount out of 100; 17.6%, then, is equivalent to 17.6 out of 100, or $\frac{17.6}{100}$. A percentage can be converted into decimal form by dividing it by 100, or, more simply, by shifting the decimal point two places to the left. Therefore, 17.6% is equivalent to 0.176.

43. D: The answer is 1.26. To solve this problem, you must know how to convert percentages into decimals. Remember that a percentage is really just an expression of a value in terms of hundredths. That is, 25% is the same as 25 out of 100. To convert a percentage into a decimal, shift the decimal point two places to the left. In this case, the decimal point is assumed to be after the six in 126%. By shifting the decimal point two places to the left, you find that the equivalent decimal is 1.26.

44. C: The answer is 22%. This problem requires you to understand how to convert fractions into percentages. To do so, divide the numerator by the denominator. This requires placing a decimal point and 0 after the 2. Remember that the instructions ask you to round your quotient to the nearest whole number. The quotient will be an endlessly repeating 0.2, which means that you will round down to 22%. You only need to solve this equation to the thousandths place in order to obtain sufficient information to answer the question.

45. B: The answer is 69%. To solve this problem, you must know how to convert fractions into percentages. This is done by dividing the numerator by the denominator. In this case, the problem is set up as $13\overline{)9.0}$, because a decimal point and 0 are required to make the calculation possible. Although the decimal point is there, you should still treat 9.0 as if it were 90 when performing your division. Since 13 will go into 90 six times, you can place a 6 above the 0 in 9.0. Remember that your quotient will have a decimal point in the identical place; that is, directly to the left of the 6. If you continue your calculations, you will derive an answer of 0.692... However, once you derive that first 6, you should be able to select the correct answer choice. Remember that percentage is the same as hundredths; in other words, 69% is the same as sixty-nine hundredths.

46. B: The answer is 25%. This problem requires you to understand how to convert fractions into percentages. One way to make this conversion is to divide 17 by 68, which will create a decimal quotient, and then convert this decimal into a percentage. The procedure for division is the same as was used in problem 45; simply divide the numerator (17) by the denominator (68). In order to do so, you will have to express 17 as 17.0. Take the resulting quotient, 0.25, and convert it into a percentage by multiplying it by a hundred or simply shifting the decimal point two places to the right. Of course, you may skip this last step if your quotient makes the right answer apparent. In this problem, for instance, a quotient of 0.25 suggests that only answer choice B can be correct.

47. C: The answer is 59%. To solve this problem, you must know how to convert a fraction into a percentage. Gerald made 13 out of 22 shots, a performance that can also be expressed by the fraction 13/22. To convert this fraction into a percentage, divide the numerator by the denominator: $22\overline{)13}$. Once you derive the initial 5 in the quotient, you can be fairly certain that answer choice C is correct. Whenever possible, try to take these kinds of shortcuts to save yourself some time. Although the HESI exam gives you plenty of time to complete all of the questions, by saving a little time here and there you can give yourself more opportunities to work through the harder problems.

48. A: The answer is 108. This problem requires you to understand how to find equivalencies involving percentages. One way to solve this problem is to set up the equation $\frac{18}{100}=\frac{x}{600}$. In words, this equation states that 18 out of 100 is equal to some unknown amount out of 600. The first step in solving such an equation is to cross-multiply; in other words, 18 × 600 = 100x. This produces 10,800 = 100x, a problem that can be solved for x by dividing both sides by 100. This calculation shows that x = 108, meaning that 108 is 18% of 600.

49. D: The answer is 2.0. To solve this problem, you must know how to find equivalencies involving percentages. This problem can be solved with the same strategy used in problem 48. To begin with, set up the following equation: $\frac{6.4}{100}=\frac{x}{32}$. Next cross-multiply: 6.4 × 32 = 100x. This produces 204.8 = 100x, which is solved for x by dividing both sides of the equation by 100. The value of x is 2.048, which is rounded to 2.0.

50. B: The answer is 17. This problem requires you to know about Roman numerals. This system of numeration is still used in a number of professional contexts. The Roman numerals are as follows: I (1), V (5), X (10), L (50), C (100), D (500), and M (1000). You may also see the lowercase versions of these letters used. The order of the numerals is typically largest to smallest. However, when a smaller number is placed in front of a larger one, the smaller number is to be subtracted from the larger one that follows. For instance, the Roman numeral XIV is 14, as the 1 (I) is to be subtracted from the 5 (V). If the number had been written XVI, it would represent 16, as the 1 (I) is to be added to the 5 (V).

BiologyAnswerKeyandExplanations

1. B: It is impossible for an *AaBb* organism to have the *aa* combination in the gametes. It is impossible for each letter to be used more than one time, so it would be impossible for the lowercase *a* to appear twice in the gametes. It would be possible, however, for *Aa* to appear in the gametes, since there is one uppercase *A* and one lowercase *a*. Gametes are the cells involved in sexual reproduction. They are germ cells.

2. A: The typical result of mitosis in humans is two diploid cells. *Mitosis* is the division of a body cell into two daughter cells. Each of the two produced cells has the same set of chromosomes as the parent. A diploid cell contains both sets of homologous chromosomes. A haploid cell contains only one set of chromosomes, which means that it only has a single set of genes. For the HESI exam, you will need to know about all the different stages of cell division for both human and plant cells.

3. B: Water stabilizes the temperature of living things. The ability of warm-blooded animals, including human beings, to maintain a constant internal temperature is known as *homeostasis*. Homeostasis depends on the presence of water in the body. Water tends to minimize changes in temperature because it takes a while to heat up or cool down. When the human body gets warm, the blood vessels dilate and blood moves away from the torso and toward the extremities. When the body gets cold, blood concentrates in the torso. This is the reason why hands and feet tend to get especially cold in cold weather. The HESI exam will require you to understand the basic processes of the human body.

4. B: Oxygen is not one of the products of the Krebs cycle. The *Krebs cycle* is the second stage of cellular respiration. In this stage, a sequence of reactions converts pyruvic acid into carbon dioxide. This stage of cellular respiration produces the phosphate compounds that provide most of the energy for the cell. The Krebs cycle is also known as the citric acid cycle or the tricarboxylic acid cycle. The HESI exam may require you to know all stages of cellular respiration: the process in which a plant cell converts carbon dioxide into oxygen.

5. C: The sugar and phosphate in DNA are connected by covalent bonds. A *covalent bond* is formed when atoms share electrons. It is very common for atoms to share pairs of electrons. An *ionicbond* is created when one or more electrons are transferred between atoms. *Ionic bonds*, also known as *electrovalent bonds*, are formed between ions with opposite charges. There is no such thing as an *overt bond* in chemistry. The HESI exam will require you to understand and have some examples of these different types of bonds.

6. A: The second part of an organism's scientific name is its species. The system of naming species is called binomial nomenclature. The first name is the *genus*, and the second name is the *species*. In binomial nomenclature, species is the most specific designation. This system enables the same name to be used all around the world, so that scientists can communicate with one another. Genus and species are just two of the categories in biological classification, otherwise known as taxonomy. The levels of classification, from most general to most specific, are kingdom, phylum, class, order, family, genus, and species. As you can see, binomial nomenclature only includes the two most specific categories.

7. B: Unlike other organic molecules, lipids are not water soluble. Lipids are typically composed of carbon and hydrogen. Three common types of lipid are fats, waxes, and oils. Indeed, lipids usually feel oily when you touch them. All living cells are primarily composed of lipids, carbohydrates, and proteins. Some examples of fats are lard, corn oil, and butter. Some examples of waxes are beeswax and carnauba wax. Some examples of steroids are cholesterol and ergosterol.

8. D:*Hemoglobin* is not a steroid. It is a protein that helps to move oxygen from the lungs to the various body tissues. Steroids can be either synthetic chemicals used to reduce swelling and inflammation or sex hormones produced by the body. *Cholesterol* is the most abundant steroid in the human body. It is necessary for the creation of bile, though it can be dangerous if the levels in the body become too high. *Estrogen* is a female steroid produced by the ovaries (in females), testes (in males), placenta, and adrenal cortex. It contributes to adolescent sexual development, menstruation, mood, lactation, and aging. *Testosterone* is the main hormone produced by the testes; it is responsible for the development of adult male sex characteristics.

9. A: The property of cohesion is responsible for the passage of water through a plant. *Cohesion* is the attractive force between two molecules of the same substance. The water in the roots of the plant is drawn upward into the stem, leaves, and flowers by the presence of other water molecules. *Adhesion* is the attractive force between molecules of different substances. *Osmosis* is a process in which water diffuses through a selectively permeable membrane. *Evaporation* is the conversion of water from a liquid to a gas.

10. C:*Melatonin* is produced by the pineal gland. One of the primary functions of melatonin is regulation of the circadian cycle, which is the rhythm of sleep and wakefulness. *Insulin* helps regulate the amount of glucose in the blood. Without insulin, the body is unable to convert blood sugar into energy. *Testosterone* is the main hormone produced by the testes; it is responsible for the development of adult male sex characteristics. *Epinephrine*, also known as adrenaline, performs a number of functions: It quickens and strengthens the heartbeat and dilates the bronchioles. Epinephrine is one of the hormones secreted when the body senses danger.

11. C:*Ribosomes* are the organelles that organize protein synthesis. A ribosome, composed of RNA and protein, is a tiny structure responsible for putting proteins together. The *mitochondrion* converts chemical energy into a form that is more useful for the functions of the cell. The *nucleus* is the central structure of the cell. It contains the DNA and administrates the functions of the cell. The *vacuole* is a cell organelle in which useful materials (for example, carbohydrates, salts, water, and proteins) are stored.

12. D: During *meiosis I,* the chromosome number is reduced from diploid to haploid. *Interphase* is the period of the cell cycle that occurs in between divisions of the cell. In *meiosis*, the homologous chromosomes in a diploid cell separate, reducing the number of chromosomes in each cell by half. *Mitosis* is the phase of cell division in which the cell nucleus divides. *S phase* is the part of the mitotic cycle in which DNA is synthesized.

13. C: Prokaryotic cells do not contain a nucleus. A *prokaryote* is simply a single-celled organism without a nucleus. It is difficult to identify the structures of a prokaryotic cell, even with a microscope. These cells are usually shaped like a rod, a sphere, or a spiral. A *eukaryote* is an organism containing cells with nuclei. Bacterial cells are prokaryotes, but since there are other kinds of prokaryotes, *bacteria* cannot be the correct answer to this question. *Cancer* cells are malignant, atypical cells that reproduce to the detriment of the organism in which they are located.

14. A:*Phenotype* is the physical presentation of an organism's genes. In other words, the phenotype is the physical characteristics of the organism. Phenotype is often contrasted with *genotype*, the genetic makeup of an organism. The genotype of the organism is not visible in its presentation, although some of the characteristics encoded in the genes have to do with physical presentation. A *phylum* is a group of classes that are closely related. A *species* is a group of like organisms that are capable of breeding together and producing similar offspring.

15. A: Liquid is the densest form of water. Water can exist in three states, depending on temperature. Ranging from coldest to hottest, these states are solid, liquid, and gaseous—or ice, water, and steam. Water freezes at zero degrees Celsius. Although the solidity of ice might lead one to believe that it is the densest form of water, water actually expands about nine percent when it is frozen. This is the reason why ice will float in water. Steam is the least dense form of water.

16. B: *Interphase* is the longest phase in the life of a cell. Interphase occurs between cell divisions. *Prophase* is the initial stage of mitosis. It is also the longest stage. During prophase, the chromosomes become visible, and the centrioles divide and position themselves on either side of the nucleus. *Anaphase* is the third phase of mitosis, in which chromosome pairs divide and take up positions on opposing poles. *Metaphase* is the second stage of mitosis. In it, the chromosomes align themselves across the center of the cell.

17. A: Bacterial cells do not contain *mitochondria*. Bacteria are prokaryotes composed of single cells; their cell walls contain peptidoglycans. The functions normally performed in the mitochondria are performed in the cell membrane of the bacterial cell. *DNA* is the nucleic acid that contains the genetic information of the organism. It is in the shape of a double helix. DNA can reproduce itself and can synthesize RNA. A *vesicle* is a small cavity containing fluid. A *ribosome* is a tiny particle composed of RNA and protein, in which polypeptides are constructed.

18. B: *Hemoglobin* is a protein. Proteins contain carbon, nitrogen, oxygen, and hydrogen. These substances are required for the growth and repair of tissue and the formation of enzymes. Hemoglobin is found in red blood cells and contains iron. It is responsible for carrying oxygen from the lungs to the various body tissues. *Adenosine triphosphate* (ATP) is a compound used by living organisms to store and use energy. *Estrogen* is a steroid hormone that stimulates the development of female sex characteristics. *Cellulose* is a complex carbohydrate that composes the better part of the cell wall.

19. D: Deoxyribonucleic acid (*DNA*) is not involved in translation. *Translation* is the process by which messenger RNA (*mRNA*) messages are decoded into polypeptide chains. Transfer RNA (*tRNA*) is a molecule that moves amino acids into the ribosomes during the synthesis of protein. Messenger RNA carries sets of instructions for the conversion of amino acids into proteins from the RNA to the other parts of the cell. *Ribosomes* are the tiny particles in the cell where proteins are put together. Ribosomes are composed of ribonucleic acid (RNA) and protein.

20. A: Water is required for cell diffusion. Diffusion is the movement of molecules from an area of high concentration to an area of lower concentration. This process takes place in the body in a number of different areas. For instance, nutrients diffuse from partially digested food through the walls of the intestine into the bloodstream. Similarly, oxygen that enters the lungs diffuses into the bloodstream through membranes at the end of the alveoli. In all these cases, the body has evolved special membranes that only allow certain materials through.

21. C: There are four different nucleotides in DNA. *Nucleotides* are monomers of nucleic acids, composed of five-carbon sugars, a phosphate group, and a nitrogenous base. Nucleotides make up both DNA and RNA. They are essential for the recording of an organism's genetic information, which guides the actions of the various cells of the body. Nucleotides are also a crucial component of adenosine triphosphate (ATP), one of the parts of DNA and a chemical that enables metabolism and muscle contractions.

22. B: *Red blood cells* do not have a nucleus. These cells are shaped a little like a doughnut, although the hole in the center is not quite open. The other three types of cell have a nucleus. *Platelets*, which are fragments of cells and are released by the bone marrow, contribute to blood clotting. *White* *blood cells*, otherwise known as leukocytes, help the body fight disease. A *phagocyte* is a cell that can entirely surround bacteria and other microorganisms. The two most common phagocytes are neutrophils and monocytes, both of which are white blood cells.

23. D: The *electrontransport system* enacted during aerobic respiration requires oxygen. This is the last component of biological oxidation. *Osmosis* is the movement of fluid from an area of high concentration through a partially permeable membrane to an area of lower concentration. This process usually stops when the concentration is the same on either side of the membrane. *Glycolysis* is the initial step in the release of glucose energy. The *Krebs cycle* is the last phase of the process in which cells convert food into energy. It is during this stage that carbon dioxide is produced and hydrogen is extracted from molecules of carbon.

24. A:*Kingdom* is the largest, most expansive taxonomic category. A *genus* is a group of related species, which are capable of breeding and producing similar offspring. In binomial nomenclature, genus is the first name. An *order* is any group of similar families. A *phylum* is any group of closely related classes. The HESI exam requires you to know the name and relative specificity of each taxonomic category. They are listed here in order from most general to most specific: kingdom, phylum, class, order, family, genus, and species.

25. D:*Fission* is the process of a bacterial cell splitting into two new cells. Fission is a form of asexual reproduction in which an organism divides into two components; each of these two parts will develop into a distinct organism. The two cells, known as daughter cells, are identical. *Mitosis*, on the other hand, is the part of eukaryotic cell division in which the cell nucleus divides. In *meiosis*, the homologous chromosomes in a diploid cell separate, reducing the number of chromosomes in each cell by half. In *replication*, a cell creates duplicate copies of DNA.

ChemistryAnswerKeyandExplanations

1. A: Diffusion is fastest through gases. The next fastest medium for diffusion is liquid, followed by plasma, and then solids. In chemistry, diffusion is defined as the movement of matter by the random motions of molecules. In a gas or a liquid, the molecules are in perpetual motion. For instance, in a quantity of seemingly immobile air, molecules of nitrogen and oxygen are constantly bouncing off each other. There is even some miniscule degree of diffusion in solids, which rises in proportion to the temperature of the substance.

2. B: The oxidation number of the hydrogen in CaH_2 is -1. The oxidation number is the positive or negative charge of a monoatomic ion. In other words, the oxidation number is the numerical charge on an ion. An ion is a charged version of an element. Oxidation number is often referred to as oxidation state. Oxidation number is sometimes used to describe the number of electrons that must be added or removed from an atom in order to convert the atom to its elemental form.

3. A: Boron does not exist as a diatomic molecule. The other possible answer choices, fluorine, oxygen, and nitrogen, all exist as diatomic molecules. A diatomic molecule always appears in nature as a pair: The word *diatomic* means "having two atoms." With the exception of astatine, all of the halogens are diatomic. Chemistry students often use the mnemonic BrINClHOF (pronounced "brinkelhoff") to remember all of the diatomic elements: bromine, iodine, nitrogen, chlorine, hydrogen, oxygen, and fluorine. Note that not all of these diatomic elements are halogens.

4. D: Hydriodic acid is another name for aqueous HI. In an aqueous solution, the solvent is water. Hydriodic acid is a polyatomic ion, meaning that it is composed of two or more elements. When this solution has an increased amount of oxygen, the *-ate* suffix on the first word is converted to *-ic*. The

HESI exam will require you to know the fundamentals of naming chemicals. This process can be quite complex, so you should carefully review this material before your exam.

5. C: CH could be an empirical formula. An empirical formula is the smallest expression of a chemical formula. To be empirical, a formula must be incapable of being reduced. For this reason, answer choices A, B, and D are incorrect, as they could all be reduced to a simpler form. Note that empirical formulas are not the same as compounds, which do not have to be irreducible. Two compounds can have the same empirical formula but different molecular formulas. The molecular formula is the actual number of atoms in the molecule.

6. A: A limiting reactant is entirely used up by the chemical reaction. Limiting reactants control the extent of the reaction and determine the quantity of the product. A reducing agent is a substance that reduces the amount of another substance by losing electrons. A reagent is any substance used in a chemical reaction. Some of the most common reagents in the laboratory are sodium hydroxide and hydrochloric acid. The behavior and properties of these substances are known, so they can be effectively used to produce predictable reactions in an experiment.

7. B: The horizontal rows of the periodic table are called periods. The vertical columns of the periodic table are known as groups or families. All of the elements in a group have similar properties. The relationships between the elements in each period are similar as you move from left to right. The periodic table was developed by Dmitri Mendeleev to organize the known elements according to their similarities. New elements can be added to the periodic table without necessitating a redesign.

8. C: The mass of 7.35 mol water is 132 grams. You should be able to find the mass of various chemical compounds when you are given the number of mols. The information required to perform this function is included on the periodic table. To solve this problem, find the molecular mass of water by finding the respective weights of hydrogen and oxygen. Remember that water contains two hydrogen molecules and one oxygen molecule. The molecular mass of hydrogen is roughly 1, and the molecular mass of oxygen is roughly 16. A molecule of water, then, has approximately 18 grams of mass. Multiply this by 7.35 mol, and you will obtain the answer 132.3, which is closest to answer choice C.

9. D: Of these orbitals, the last to fill is 6s. Orbitals fill in the following order: 1s, 2s, 2p, 3s, 3p, 4s, 3d, 4p, 5s, 4d, 5p, 6s, 4f, 5d, 6p, 7s, 5f, 6d, and 7p. The number is the orbital number, and the letter is the sublevel identification. Sublevel s has one orbital and can hold a maximum of two electrons. Sublevel p has three orbitals and can hold a maximum of six electrons. Sublevel d has five orbitals and can hold a maximum of 10 electrons. Sublevel f has seven orbitals and can hold a maximum of 14 electrons.

10. C: Nitrogen pentoxide is the name of the binary molecular compound NO_5. The format given in answer choice C is appropriate when dealing with two nonmetals. A prefix is used to denote the number of atoms of each element. Note that when there are seven atoms of a given element, the prefix *hepta-* is used instead of the usual *septa-*. Also, when the first atom in this kind of binary molecular compound is single, it does not need to be given the prefix *mono-*.

11. D: The mass of 1.0 mol oxygen gas is 32 grams. The molar mass of oxygen can be obtained from the periodic table. In most versions of the table, the molar mass of the element is directly beneath the full name of the element. There is a little trick to this question. Oxygen is a diatomic molecule, which means that it always appears in pairs. In order to determine the mass in grams of 1.0 mol of oxygen gas, then, you must double the molar mass. The listed mass is 16, so the correct answer to the problem is 32.

12. D: Gamma radiation has no charge. This form of electromagnetic radiation can travel a long distance and can penetrate the human body. Sunlight and radio waves are both examples of gamma radiation. Alpha radiation has a 2+ charge. It only travels short distances and cannot penetrate clothing or skin. Radium and uranium both emit alpha radiation. Beta radiation has a 1– charge. It can travel several feet through the air and is capable of penetrating the skin. This kind of radiation can be damaging to health over a long period of exposure. There is no such thing as delta radiation.

13. A: When forward and reverse chemical reactions are taking place at the same rate, a chemical reaction has achieved equilibrium. This means that the respective concentrations of reactants and products do not change over time. In theory, a chemical reaction will remain in equilibrium indefinitely. One of the common tasks in the chemistry lab is to find the equilibrium constant (or set of relative concentrations that result in equilibrium) for a given reaction. In thermal equilibrium, there is no net heat exchange between a body and its surroundings. In dynamic equilibrium, any motion in one direction is offset by an equal motion in the other direction.

14. B: 119°K is equivalent to –154 degrees Celsius. It is likely that you will have to perform at least one temperature conversion on the HESI exam. To convert degrees Kelvin to degrees Celsius, simply subtract 273. To convert degrees Celsius to degrees Kelvin, simply add 273. To convert degrees Kelvin into degrees Fahrenheit, multiply by 9/5 and subtract 460. To convert degrees Fahrenheit to degrees Kelvin, add 460 and then multiply by 5/9. To convert degrees Celsius to degrees Fahrenheit, multiply by 9/5 and then add 32. To convert degrees Fahrenheit to degrees Celsius, subtract 32 and then multiply by 5/9.

15. B: The *joule* is the SI unit of energy. Energy is the ability to do work or generate heat. In regard to electrical energy, a joule is the amount of electrical energy required to pass a current of one ampere through a resistance of one ohm for one second. In physical or mechanical terms, the joule is the amount of energy required for a force of one newton to act over a distance of one meter. The *ohm* is a unit of electrical resistance. The *henry* is a unit of inductance. The *newton* is a unit of force.

16. A: A *mass spectrometer* separates gaseous ions according to their mass-to-charge ratio. This machine is used to distinguish the various elements in a piece of matter. An *interferometer* measures the wavelength of light by comparing the interference phenomena of two waves: an experimental wave and a reference wave. A *magnetometer* measures the direction and magnitude of a magnetic field. Finally, a *capacitance meter* measures the capacitance of a capacitor. Some sophisticated capacitance meters may also measure inductance, leakage, and equivalent series resistance.

17. C: Of the given materials, aluminum has the smallest specific heat. The specific heat of a substance is the amount of heat required to raise the temperature of one gram of the substance by one degree Celsius. In some cases, specific heat is expressed as a ratio of the heat required to raise the temperature of one gram of a substance by one degree Celsius to the heat required to raise the temperature of one gram of water by one degree Celsius.

18. C: In a *redox* reaction, also known as an oxidation-reduction reaction, electrons are transferred from one atom to another. A redox reaction changes the oxidation numbers of the atoms. In a *combustion* reaction, one material combines with an oxidizer to form a product and generate heat. In a *synthesis* reaction, multiple chemicals are combined to create a more complex product. In a *double-displacement* reaction, two chemical compounds trade bonds or ions and create two different compounds. Other common chemical reactions you may need to know for the HESI exam are the acid-base reaction, analysis reaction, single-displacement reaction, isomerization reaction, and hydrolysis reaction.

19. A: Van der Waals forces are the weak forces of attraction between two molecules. The van der Waals force is considered to be any of the attractive or repulsive forces between electrons that are not related to electrostatic interaction or covalent bonds. Compared to other chemical bonds, the strength of van der Waals forces is small. However, these forces have a great effect on a substance's solubility and other characteristics. The HESI exam may require you to demonstrate knowledge of all the major chemical forces.

20. D: Of the given gases, H_2 effuses the fastest. It has the smallest molecular weight, and it is therefore capable of moving faster than the molecules represented by the other answer choices. In chemistry, effusion is defined as the flow of a gas through a small opening. The rate of effusion of a substance is inversely proportional to the square root of the density of the substance. This means that the less dense a substance is, the faster it will effuse. This agrees with the common observation that thick smoke tends to linger in the same form for a longer period than thin smoke or steam.

21. B: Carbon is not involved in many hydrogen bonds. A hydrogen bond occurs when an atom of hydrogen that has a covalent bond with an electronegative atom forms a bond with a third atom. The original covalent bond involving hydrogen gives away protons, and the third element receives them. One of the reasons that fluorine, oxygen, and nitrogen are frequently part of a hydrogen bond is that they have a strong electronegativity and are therefore able to form more durable bonds. Chlorine is another element frequently involved in hydrogen bonds.

22. D: The mass of 0.350 mol copper is 22.2 grams. This problem requires the use of the periodic table. There you will see that the molecular mass of copper is approximately 63.5. Take this figure and multiply it by the amount of copper given by the question: 0.350 mol. The resulting figure is 22.225, which, rounded to the nearest tenth, is 22.2 grams. In order to succeed on the HESI exam, you will need to be able to perform these simple calculations of mass.

23. A: There are five d orbitals in a d subshell (or sublevel). Each of these orbitals can hold two electrons, so sublevel d is capable of holding 10 electrons. The s subshell has one orbital, the p subshell has three orbitals, the d subshell has five orbitals, and the f subshell has seven orbitals. In chemistry, the electron configuration of an atom is expressed in the following form, using helium as an example: $1s^2$. In this notation, the 1 indicates that the electrons are found in the first energy level of the atom, the s indicates that the electrons are in a spherical orbit, and the superscript 2 indicates that there are 2 total electrons in the first energy level subshell.

24. D: The number of protons in an atom is the atomic number. Protons are the fundamental positive unit of an atom. They are located in the nucleus. In a neutral atom (an atom with neither positive nor negative charge), the number of protons in the nucleus is equal to the number of electrons orbiting the nucleus. When it needs to be expressed, atomic number is written as a subscript in front of the element's symbol, for example in $_{13}Al$. Atomic mass, meanwhile, is the average mass of the various isotopes of a given element. Atomic identity and atomic weight are not concepts in chemistry.

25. B: Rubidium is an alkali metal. The alkali metals are located in group 1 of the periodic table. These soft substances melt at a low temperature and are typically white in color. The alkali metals are lithium, sodium, potassium, rubidium, cesium, and francium. Rubidium, cesium, and francium are not commonly encountered in the natural world. The alkali metals are highly reactive, meaning that they easily engage in chemical reactions when combined with other elements. These metals have a low density and tend to react violently with water.

AnatomyandPhysiologyAnswerKeyandExplanations

1. D: The epiglottis covers the trachea during swallowing, thus preventing food from entering the airway. The trachea, also known as the windpipe, is a cylindrical portion of the respiratory tract that joins the larynx with the lungs. The esophagus connects the throat and the stomach. When a person swallows, the esophagus contracts to force the food down into the stomach. Like other structures in the respiratory system, the esophagus secretes mucus for lubrication.

2. B: The pads that support the vertebrae are made up of cartilage. Cartilage, a strong form of connective tissue, cushions and supports the joints. Cartilage also makes up the larynx and the outer ear. Bone is a form of connective tissue that comprises the better part of the skeleton. It includes both organic and inorganic substances. Tendons connect the muscles to other structures of the body, typically bones. Tendons can increase and decrease in length as the bones move. Fat is a combination of lipids; in humans, fat forms a layer beneath the skin and on the outside of the internal organs.

3. A: There are four different types of tissue in the human body: epithelial, connective, muscle, and nerve. *Epithelial* tissue lines the internal and external surfaces of the body. It is like a sheet, consisting of squamous, cuboidal, and columnar cells. They can expand and contract, like on the inner lining of the bladder. *Connective* tissue provides the structure of the body, as well as the links between various body parts. Tendons, ligaments, cartilage, and bone are all examples of connective tissue. *Muscle* tissue is composed of tiny fibers, which contract to move the skeleton. There are three types of muscle tissue: smooth, cardiac, and skeletal. *Nerve* tissue makes up the nervous system; it is composed of nerve cells, nerve fibers, neuroglia, and dendrites.

4. B: The epidermis is the outermost layer of skin. The thickness of this layer of skin varies over different parts of the body. For instance, the epidermis on the eyelids is very thin, while the epidermis over the soles of the feet is much thicker. The dermis lies directly beneath the epidermis. It is composed of collagen, elastic tissue, and reticular fibers. Beneath the dermis lies the subcutaneous tissue, which consists of fat, blood vessels, and nerves. The subcutaneous tissue contributes to the regulation of body temperature. The hypodermis is the layer of cells underneath the dermis; it is generally considered to be a part of the subcutaneous tissue.

5. C:*Prolactin* stimulates the production of breast milk during lactation. *Norepinephrine* is a hormone and neurotransmitter secreted by the adrenal gland that regulates heart rate, blood pressure, and blood sugar. *Antidiuretic hormone* is produced by the hypothalamus and secreted by the pituitary gland. It regulates the concentration of urine and triggers the contractions of the arteries and capillaries. *Oxytocin* is a hormone secreted by the pituitary gland that makes it easier to eject milk from the breast and manages the contractions of the uterus during labor.

6. D: Of the given structures, veins have the lowest blood pressure. *Veins* carry oxygen-poor blood from the outlying parts of the body to the heart. An *artery* carries oxygen-rich blood from the heart to the peripheral parts of the body. An *arteriole* extends from an artery to a capillary. A *venule* is a tiny vein that extends from a capillary to a larger vein.

7. C: Of the four heart chambers, the left ventricle is the most muscular. When it contracts, it pushes blood out to the organs and extremities of the body. The right ventricle pushes blood into the lungs. The atria, on the other hand, receive blood from the outlying parts of the body and transport it into the ventricles. The basic process works as follows: Oxygen-poor blood fills the right atrium and is pumped into the right ventricle, from which it is pumped into the pulmonary artery and on to the lungs. In the lungs, this blood is oxygenated. The blood then reenters the heart at the left atrium, which when full pumps into the left ventricle. When the left ventricle is full, blood is pushed into the aorta and on to the organs and extremities of the body.

8. A: The *cerebrum* is the part of the brain that interprets sensory information. It is the largest part of the brain. The cerebrum is divided into two hemispheres, connected by a thin band of tissue called the corpus callosum. The *cerebellum* is positioned at the back of the head, between the brain stem and the cerebrum. It controls both voluntary and involuntary movements. The *medulla oblongata* forms the base of the brain. This part of the brain is responsible for blood flow and breathing, among other things.

9. C:*Collagen* is the protein produced by cartilage. Bone, tendon, and cartilage are all mainly composed of collagen. *Actin* and *myosin* are the proteins responsible for muscle contractions. Actin makes up the thinner fibers in muscle tissue, while myosin makes up the thicker fibers. Myosin is the most numerous cell protein in human muscle. *Estrogen* is one of the steroid hormones produced mainly by the ovaries. Estrogen motivates the menstrual cycle and the development of female sex characteristics.

10. C: The parasympathetic nervous system is responsible for lowering the heart rate. It slows down the heart rate, dilates the blood vessels, and increases the secretions of the digestive system. The central nervous system is composed of the brain and the spinal cord. The sympathetic nervous system is a part of the autonomic nervous system; its role is to oppose the actions taken by the parasympathetic nervous system. So, the sympathetic nervous system accelerates the heart, contracts the blood vessels, and decreases the secretions of the digestive system.

11. B: Urea is formed during the breakdown of proteins. It is a nitrogen-rich substance filtered out of the bloodstream by the kidneys and expelled from the body in the urine. Individuals with an elevated level of urea in their bloodstream may be suffering from kidney failure. In humans and most animals, urea is the primary component of urine. However, urine also contains uric acid and ammonia. Both of these substances can be toxic to humans if they are not expelled from the body. This is one of the dangers of kidney disease and kidney failure.

12. A: A hinge joint can only move in two directions. The elbow is a hinge joint. It can only bring the lower arm closer to the upper arm or move it away from the upper arm. In a ball-and-socket joint, the rounded top of one bone fits into a concave part of another bone, enabling the first bone to rotate around in this socket. This connection is slightly less stable than other types of joints in the human body and is therefore supported by a denser network of ligaments. The shoulder and hip are both examples of ball-and-socket joints.

13. B: Smooth muscle tissue is said to be arranged in a disorderly fashion because it is not striated like the other two types of muscle: cardiac and skeletal. Striations are lines that can only be seen with a microscope. *Smooth* muscle is typically found in the supporting tissues of hollow organs and blood vessels. *Cardiac* muscle is found exclusively in the heart; it is responsible for the contractions that pump blood throughout the body. *Skeletal* muscle, by far the most preponderant in the body, controls the movements of the skeleton. The contractions of skeletal muscle are responsible for all voluntary motion. There is no such thing as *rough* muscle.

14. A: An adult inhales 500 mL of air in an average breath. Interestingly, humans can inhale about eight times as much air in a single breath as they do in an average breath. People tend to take a larger breath after making a larger inhalation. This is one reason that many breathing therapies, for instance those incorporated into yoga practice, focus on making a complete exhalation. The process of respiration is managed by the autonomic nervous system. The body requires a constant replenishing of oxygen, so even brief interruptions in respiration can be damaging or fatal.

3 HESI Admission Assessment Practice Tests

15. D:*Plasma* cells secrete antibodies. These cells, also known as plasmacytes, are located in lymphoid tissue. Antibodies are only secreted in response to a particular stimulus, usually the detection of an antigen in the body. Antigens include bacteria, viruses, and parasites. Once released, antibodies bind to the antigen and neutralize it. When faced with a new antigen, the body may require some time to develop appropriate antibodies. Once the body has learned about an antigen, however, it does not forget how to produce the correct antibodies.

16. D: The force of *blood pressure* motivates filtration in the kidneys. *Filtration* is the process through which the kidneys remove waste products from the body. All of the water in the blood passes through the kidneys every 45 minutes. Waste products are diverted into ducts and excreted from the body, while the healthy components of the water in blood are reabsorbed into the bloodstream. *Peristalsis* is the set of involuntary muscle movements that move food through the digestive system.

17. A:*Insulin* decreases the concentration of blood glucose. It is produced by the pancreas. *Glucagon* is a hormone produced by the pancreas. Glucagon acts in opposition to insulin, motivating an increase in the levels of blood sugar. *Growth hormone* is secreted by the pituitary gland. It is responsible for the growth of the body, specifically by metabolizing proteins, carbohydrates, and lipids. The *glucocorticoids* are a group of steroid hormones that are produced by the adrenal cortex. The glucocorticoids contribute to the metabolism of carbohydrates, proteins, and fats.

18. A: The *hypothalamus* controls the hormones secreted by the pituitary gland. This part of the brain maintains the body temperature and helps to control metabolism. The *adrenal glands*, which lie above the kidneys, secrete steroidal hormones, epinephrine, and norepinephrine. The *testes* are the male reproductive glands, responsible for the production of sperm and testosterone. The *pancreas* secretes insulin and a fluid that aids in digestion.

19. C: Forty percent of female blood volume is composed of red blood cells. Red blood cells, otherwise known as erythrocytes, are large and do not have a nucleus. These cells are produced in the bone marrow and carry oxygen throughout the body. White blood cells, also known as leukocytes, make up about 1% of the blood volume. About 55% of the blood volume is made up of plasma, which itself is primarily composed of water. The plasma in blood supplies cells with nutrients and removes metabolic waste. Blood also contains platelets, otherwise known as thrombocytes, which are essential to effective blood clotting.

20. B: High-density lipoproteins (*HDL*) are considered to be the healthiest form of cholesterol. This type of cholesterol actually reduces the risk of heart disease. A lipoprotein is composed of both lipid and protein. These substances cannot move through the bloodstream by themselves; they must be carried along by some other substance. Although most people think of cholesterol as an unhealthy substance, it helps to maintain cell walls and produce hormones. Cholesterol is also important in the production of vitamin D and the bile acids that aid digestion. The other answer choices are low-density lipoproteins (*LDL*), very-low-density lipoproteins (*VLDL*), and very-high-density lipoproteins (*VHDL*).

21. C: The vocal cords are located in the larynx. These elastic bands vibrate and produce sound when air passes through them. The *larynx* lies between the pharynx and the trachea. The pharynx is the section of the throat that extends from the mouth and the nasal cavities to the larynx, at which point it becomes the esophagus. The *trachea* is the tube running from the larynx down to the lungs, where it terminates in the *bronchi*. The *epiglottis* is the flap that blocks food from the lungs by descending over the trachea during a swallow.

22. A: Gas exchange occurs in the *alveoli*, the minute air sacs on the interior of the lungs. The *bronchi* are large cartilage-based tubes of air; they extend from the end of the trachea into the lungs, where they branch apart. The *larynx*, which houses the vocal cords, is positioned between the trachea and the pharynx; it is involved in swallowing, breathing, and speaking. The *pharynx* extends from the nose to the uppermost portions of the trachea and esophagus. In order to enter these two structures, air and other matter must pass through the pharynx.

23. B:*Axons* carry action potential in the direction of synapses. Axons are the long, fiberlike structures that carry information from neurons. Electrical impulses travel along the body of the axons, some of which are up to a foot long. A *neuron* is a type of cell that is responsible for sending information throughout the body. There are several types of neurons, including muscle neurons, which respond to instructions for movement; sensory neurons, which transmit information about the external world; and interneurons, which relay messages between neurons. *Myelin* is a fat that coats the nerves and ensures the accurate transmission of information in the nervous system.

24. A: The parathyroid gland is located in the neck, directly behind the thyroid gland. It is responsible for the metabolism of calcium. It is part of the endocrine system. When the supply of calcium in blood diminishes to unhealthy levels, the parathyroid gland motivates the secretion of a hormone that encourages the bones to release calcium into the bloodstream. The parathyroid gland also regulates the amount of phosphate in the blood by stimulating the excretion of phosphates in the urine.

25. B: In the lungs, oxygen is transported from the air to the blood through the process of *diffusion*. Specifically, the alveolar membranes withdraw the oxygen from the air in the lungs into the bloodstream. *Osmosis* is the movement of a solution from an area of low concentration to an area of higher concentration through a permeable membrane. *Dissipation* is any wasteful consumption or use. *Reverse osmosis* is a process for purifying a solution by forcing it through a membrane that blocks only certain pollutants.

HESI A²PracticeTest #2

Reading Comprehension	Vocabulary and General Knowledge	Grammar	Mathematics

1. _____	1. _____ 49. _____	1. _____ 49. _____	1. _____ 49. _____
2. _____	2. _____ 50. _____	2. _____ 50. _____	2. _____ 50. _____
3. _____	3. _____	3. _____	3. _____
4. _____	4. _____	4. _____	4. _____
5. _____	5. _____	5. _____	5. _____
6. _____	6. _____	6. _____	6. _____
7. _____	7. _____	7. _____	7. _____
8. _____	8. _____	8. _____	8. _____
9. _____	9. _____	9. _____	9. _____
10. _____	10. _____	10. _____	10. _____
11. _____	11. _____	11. _____	11. _____
12. _____	12. _____	12. _____	12. _____
13. _____	13. _____	13. _____	13. _____
14. _____	14. _____	14. _____	14. _____
15. _____	15. _____	15. _____	15. _____
16. _____	16. _____	16. _____	16. _____
17. _____	17. _____	17. _____	17. _____
18. _____	18. _____	18. _____	18. _____
19. _____	19. _____	19. _____	19. _____
20. _____	20. _____	20. _____	20. _____
21. _____	21. _____	21. _____	21. _____
22. _____	22. _____	22. _____	22. _____
23. _____	23. _____	23. _____	23. _____
24. _____	24. _____	24. _____	24. _____
25. _____	25. _____	25. _____	25. _____
26. _____	26. _____	26. _____	26. _____
27. _____	27. _____	27. _____	27. _____
28. _____	28. _____	28. _____	28. _____
29. _____	29. _____	29. _____	29. _____
30. _____	30. _____	30. _____	30. _____
31. _____	31. _____	31. _____	31. _____
32. _____	32. _____	32. _____	32. _____
33. _____	33. _____	33. _____	33. _____
34. _____	34. _____	34. _____	34. _____
35. _____	35. _____	35. _____	35. _____
36. _____	36. _____	36. _____	36. _____
37. _____	37. _____	37. _____	37. _____
38. _____	38. _____	38. _____	38. _____
39. _____	39. _____	39. _____	39. _____
40. _____	40. _____	40. _____	40. _____
41. _____	41. _____	41. _____	41. _____
42. _____	42. _____	42. _____	42. _____
43. _____	43. _____	43. _____	43. _____
44. _____	44. _____	44. _____	44. _____
45. _____	45. _____	45. _____	45. _____
46. _____	46. _____	46. _____	46. _____
47. _____	47. _____	47. _____	47. _____
	48. _____	48. _____	48. _____

Biology	Chemistry	Anatomy and Physiology
1. _____	1. _____	1. _____
2. _____	2. _____	2. _____
3. _____	3. _____	3. _____
4. _____	4. _____	4. _____
5. _____	5. _____	5. _____
6. _____	6. _____	6. _____
7. _____	7. _____	7. _____
8. _____	8. _____	8. _____
9. _____	9. _____	9. _____
10. _____	10. _____	10. _____
11. _____	11. _____	11. _____
12. _____	12. _____	12. _____
13. _____	13. _____	13. _____
14. _____	14. _____	14. _____
15. _____	15. _____	15. _____
16. _____	16. _____	16. _____
17. _____	17. _____	17. _____
18. _____	18. _____	18. _____
19. _____	19. _____	19. _____
20. _____	20. _____	20. _____
21. _____	21. _____	21. _____
22. _____	22. _____	22. _____
23. _____	23. _____	23. _____
24. _____	24. _____	24. _____
25. _____	25. _____	25. _____

| Section 1. Reading Comprehension | Number of Questions: **47** |
| | Time Limit: **50 Minutes** |

Questions 1 to 8 pertain to the following passage:

Visual Perception

It is tempting to think that your eyes are simply mirrors that reflect whatever is in front of them. Researchers, however, have shown that your brain is constantly working to create the impression of a continuous, uninterrupted world.

For instance, in the last ten minutes, you have blinked your eyes around 200 times. You have probably not been aware of any of these interruptions in your visual world. Something you probably have not seen in a long time without the aid of a mirror is your nose. It is always right there, down in the bottom corner of your vision, but your brain filters it out so that you are not aware of your nose unless you purposefully look at it.

Nor are you aware of the artery that runs right down the middle of your retina. It creates a large blind spot in your visual field, but you never notice the hole it leaves. To see this blind spot, try the following: Cover your left eye with your hand. With your right eye, look at the O on the left. As you move your head closer to the O, the X will disappear as it enters the blind spot caused by your optical nerve.

O   X

Your brain works hard to make the world look continuous!

1. The word <u>filters</u>, as used in this passage, most nearly means:
   A. Alternates
   B. Reverses
   C. Ignores
   D. Depends

2. The word <u>retina</u>, as used in this passage, most nearly means:
   A. Optical illusion
   B. Part of the eye
   C. Pattern
   D. Blindness

3. Which of the following statements can be inferred from this passage?
   A. Not all animals' brains filter out information
   B. Visual perception is not a passive process
   C. Blind spots cause accidents
   D. The eyes never reflect reality

4. What is the author's purpose for including the two letters in the middle of the passage?
    A. To demonstrate the blind spot in the visual field
    B. To organize the passage
    C. To transition between the last two paragraphs of the passage
    D. To prove that the blind spot is not real

5. What is the main purpose of this passage?
    A. To persuade the reader to pay close attention to blind spots
    B. To explain the way visual perception works
    C. To persuade the reader to consult an optometrist if the O and X disappear
    D. To prove that vision is a passive process

6. Based on the passage, which of the following statements is true?
    A. The brain cannot accurately reflect reality
    B. Glasses correct the blind spot caused by the optical nerve
    C. Vision is the least important sense
    D. The brain fills in gaps in the visual field

7. The author mentions the nose to illustrate what point?
    A. The brain filters out some visual information
    B. Not all senses work the same way
    C. Perception is a passive process
    D. The sense of smell filters out information

8. Which of the following statements can be inferred from the second paragraph?
    A. The brain filters out the sound created by the shape of the ears
    B. The brain does not perceive all activity in the visual field
    C. Closing one eye affects depth perception
    D. The brain evolved as a result of environmental factors

Questions 9 to 17 pertain to the following passage:
Oppositional Defiant Disorder
On a bad day, have you ever been irritable? Have you ever used a harsh tone or even been verbally disrespectful to your parents or teachers? Everyone has a short temper from time to time, but current statistics indicate that between 16% and 20% of a school's population suffer from a psychological condition known as Oppositional Defiance Disorder, or ODD.

ODD symptoms include difficulty complying with adult requests, excessive arguments with adults, temper tantrums, difficulty accepting responsibility for actions, low frustration tolerance, and behaviors intended to annoy or upset adults. Parents of children with ODD can often feel as though their whole relationship is based on conflict after conflict.

Unfortunately, ODD can be caused by a number of factors. Some students affected by ODD suffer abuse, neglect, and severe or unpredictable discipline at home. Others have parents with mood disorders or have experienced family violence. Various types of therapy are helpful in treating ODD, and some drugs can treat particular symptoms. However, no single cure exists.
The best advice from professionals is directed toward parents. Therapists encourage parents to avoid situations that usually end in power struggles, to try not to feed into oppositional behavior by reacting emotionally, to praise positive

behaviors, and to discourage negative behaviors with timeouts instead of harsh discipline.

9. Which of the following statements can be inferred from paragraph 4?
    A. Parents of children with ODD are bad parents
    B. ODD is not a real psychological disorder
    C. Medication can worsen ODD
    D. Reacting emotionally to defiant behavior might worsen the behavior

10. Which of the following best describes the main idea of this passage?
    A. ODD has no cause
    B. ODD is a complex condition
    C. Parents with ODD should seek support
    D. Parents are the cause of ODD

11. As used in this passage, the word oppositional most nearly means:
    A. Uncooperative
    B. Violent
    C. Passive aggressive
    D. Altruistic

12. Which of the following can be inferred from paragraph one?
    A. Most children who speak harshly to their parents have ODD
    B. Most people exhibit symptoms of ODD occasionally
    C. Between 16% and 20% of the school population has been abused
    D. A short temper is a symptom of obsessive compulsive disorder

13. As used in this passage, the phrase feed into most nearly means:
    A. Discourage
    B. Ignore
    C. Encourage
    D. Abuse

14. As used in this passage, the phrase low frustration tolerance most nearly means:
    A. Patience
    B. Low IQ
    C. Difficulty dealing with frustration
    D. The ability to cope with frustration

15. The author's purpose in writing this passage is to:
    A. Express frustration about ODD
    B. Prove that parents are the cause of ODD
    C. Inform the reader about this complex condition
    D. Persuade the reader to keep students with ODD out of public school

16. According to the passage, which of the following is a cause of ODD?
    A. Excessive television viewing
    B. Poor diet
    C. Severe or unpredictable punishment
    D. Low IQ

17. Based on the passage, which of the following statements seems most true?
    A. A variety of parenting techniques can be used to help children with ODD
    B. Children with ODD must be physically aggressive to be diagnosed
    C. Parents of children with ODD often engage in risk-taking activities
    D. Harsh disciplinary measures must be used to control children with ODD

Questions 18 to 21 pertain to the following passage:

Protozoa are microscopic, one-celled organisms that can be free-living or parasitic in nature. They are able to multiply in humans, a factor which contributes to their survival and also permits serious infections to develop from just a single organism. Transmission of protozoa that live in the human intestine to another human typically occurs by a fecal-oral route (for example, contaminated food or water, or person-to-person contact). Protozoa that thrive in the blood or tissue of humans are transmitted to their human hosts by an arthropod vector (for example, through the bite of a mosquito or sand fly).

Helminths are large, multicellular organisms that are generally visible to the naked eye in their adult stages. Like protozoa, helminths can be either free-living or parasitic in nature. In their adult form, helminths cannot multiply in humans. There are three main groups of helminths (derived from the Greek word for worms) that are human parasites:

- *Flatworms* (platyhelminths) – these include the trematodes (flukes) and cestodes (tapeworms)
- *Thorny-headed worms* (acanthocephalins) – the adult forms of these worms reside in the gastrointestinal tract. The acanthocephala are thought to be intermediate between the cestodes and nematodes
- *Roundworms* (nematodes) – the adult forms of these worms can reside in the gastrointestinal tract, blood, lymphatic system or subcutaneous tissues. Alternatively, the immature (larval) states can cause disease through their infection of various body tissues

18. As used in this passage, the word "parasite" means:
    A. A person who lives in Paris
    B. An organism that live on or in another organism
    C. Microscopic insects
    D. A person who takes advantage of the generosity of others

19. According to the passage, adult Roundworms can live in:
    A. the arthropod vector
    B. fecal matter
    C. the subcutaneous tissue of humans
    D. contaminated water

20. You can infer from this passage that:
    A. larval stages of parasites are more dangerous than the adult forms
    B. mosquitoes do not transmit parasites
    C. worms cannot infect humans
    D. clean sanitary conditions will keep you free of protozoa

21. According to the passage, which of the following is true?
  I. Protozoa live in the blood or tissue of humans
  II. Adult helminthes cannot reproduce in humans
  III. Adult Thorny-headed worms live in the intestinal tract
  A. I only
  B. II only
  C. I and II only
  D. I, II, and III

Questions 22 to 24 pertain to the following passage:
  About 17 million children and adults in the United States suffer from asthma, a condition that makes it hard to breathe. Today it is a problem that is treatable with modern medicine. In days gone by, there were many different superstitions about how to cure asthma. Some people thought that eating crickets with a little wine would help. Eating raw cat's meat might be the cure. Another idea was to try gathering some spiders' webs, rolling them into a ball, and then swallowing them. People also thought that if you ate a diet of only boiled carrots for two weeks, your asthma might go away. This carrot diet may have done some good for asthma patients since vitamin A in carrots is good for the lungs.

22. Which of the following would be a good title for the passage?
  A. Asthma in the United States
  B. Methods of treating asthma
  C. Old wives' tales
  D. Superstitions about asthma

23. The fact that 17 million children and adults in the United States suffer from asthma is probably the opening sentence of the passage because:
  A. It explains why people in times gone by might have found a need to try homemade cures
  B. It creates a contrast between today and the past
  C. It lets the reader know that many people have asthma
  D. It is a warning that anyone could get asthma

24. The main purpose of the passage is to:
  A. Describe herbal remedies
  B. Explain some of the measures for treating asthma from long ago
  C. Define superstitions
  D. Extol the virtues of modern medicine

Questions 25 and 26 pertain to the following passage:
  During the last 100 years of medical science, the drugs that have been developed have altered the way people live all over the world. Over-the-counter and prescription drugs are now the key for dealing with diseases, bodily harm, and medical issues. Drugs like these are used to add longevity and quality to people's lives. But not all drugs are healthy for every person. A drug does not necessarily have to be illegal to be abused or misused. Some ways that drugs are misused include taking more or less of the drug than is needed, using a drug that is meant for another person, taking a drug for longer than needed, taking two or more drugs at a time, or using a drug for a reason that has nothing to do with being healthy. Thousands of people die from drug misuse or abuse every year in the United States.

25. According to the passage, which of the following is an example of misusing a drug?
    A. Taking more of a prescription drug than the doctor ordered
    B. Taking an antibiotic to kill harmful bacteria
    C. Experiencing a side effect from an over-the-counter drug
    D. Throwing away a medication that has passed the expiration date

26. According to the passage, which of the following is not true?
    A. Over-the-counter drugs are used for medical issues
    B. Every year, thousands of people in the United States die due to using drugs the wrong way
    C. Medical science has come a long way in the last century
    D. All drugs add longevity to a person's life

Questions 27 to 33 pertain to the following passage:

Peanut allergy is the most prevalent food allergy in the United States, affecting around one and a half million people, and it is potentially on the rise in children in the United States. While thought to be the most common cause of food-related death, deaths from food allergies are very rare. The allergy typically begins at a very young age and remains present for life for most people. Approximately one-fifth to one-quarter of children with a peanut allergy, however, outgrow it. Treatment involves careful avoidance of peanuts or any food that may contain peanut pieces or oils. For some sufferers, exposure to even the smallest amount of peanut product can trigger a serious reaction.

Symptoms of peanut allergy can include skin reactions, itching around the mouth, digestive problems, shortness of breath, and runny or stuffy nose. The most severe peanut allergies can result in anaphylaxis, which requires immediate treatment with epinephrine. Up to one-third of people with peanut allergies have severe reactions. Without treatment, anaphylactic shock can result in death due to obstruction of the airway, or heart failure. Signs of anaphylaxis include constriction of airways and difficulty breathing, shock, a rapid pulse, and dizziness or lightheadedness.

As of yet, there is no treatment to prevent or cure allergic reactions to peanuts. In May of 2008, however, Duke University Medical Center food allergy experts announced that they expect to offer a treatment for peanut allergies within five years.

Scientists do not know for sure why peanut proteins induce allergic reactions, nor do they know why some people develop peanut allergies while others do not. There is a strong genetic component to allergies: if one of a child's parents has an allergy, the child has an almost 50% chance of developing an allergy. If both parents have an allergy, the odds increase to about 70%.
Someone suffering from a peanut allergy needs to be cautious about the foods he or she eats and the products he or she puts on his or her skin. Common foods that should be checked for peanut content are ground nuts, cereals, granola, grain breads, energy bars, and salad dressings. Store prepared cookies, pastries, and frozen desserts like ice cream can also contain peanuts. Additionally, many cuisines use peanuts in cooking – watch for peanut content in African, Chinese, Indonesian, Mexican, Thai, and Vietnamese dishes.

Parents of children with peanut allergies should notify key people (child care providers, school personnel, etc.) that their child has a peanut allergy, explain peanut allergy symptoms to them, make sure that the child's epinephrine auto injector is always available, write an action plan of care for their child when he or she has an allergic reaction to peanuts, have their child wear a medical alert bracelet or necklace, and discourage their child from sharing foods.

27. According to the passage, approximately what percentage of people with peanut allergies have severe reactions?
   A. Up to 11%
   B. Up to 22%
   C. Up to 33%
   D. Up to 55%

28. By what date do Duke University allergy experts expect to offer a treatment for peanut allergies?
   A. 2008
   B. 2009
   C. 2010
   D. 2012

29. Which of the following is not a type of cuisine the passage suggests often contains peanuts?
   A. African
   B. Italian
   C. Vietnamese
   D. Mexican

30. Which allergy does the article state is thought to be the most common cause of food-related death?
   A. Peanut
   B. Tree nut
   C. Bee sting
   D. Poison oak

31. It can be inferred from the passage that children with peanut allergies should be discouraged from sharing food because:
   A. Peanut allergies can be contagious
   B. People suffering from peanut allergies are more susceptible to bad hygiene
   C. Many foods contain peanut content and it is important to be very careful when you don't know what you're eating
   D. Scientists don't know why some people develop peanut allergies

32. Which of the following does the passage not state is a sign of anaphylaxis?
   A. Constriction of airways
   B. Shock
   C. A rapid pulse
   D. Running or stuffy nose

Questions 33 to 36 pertain to the following passage:
   Among the Atkins, South Beach and other diets people embark upon for health and weight loss is the so-called Paleolithic Diet in which adherents eat what they believe to be a diet similar to that consumed by humans during the Paleolithic era. The diet consists of food that can be hunted or gathered: primarily of meat, fish, vegetables, fruits, roots, and nuts. It does not allow for grains, legumes, dairy, salt, refined sugars or processed oils. The idea behind the diet is that humans are genetically

adapted to the diet of our Paleolithic forebears. Some studies support the idea of positive health outcomes from such a diet.

33. Which of the following does the passage not give as the name of a diet?
    A. South Beach
    B. Hunter Gatherer
    C. Paleolithic
    D. Atkins

34. Which of the following is not permitted on the Paleolithic Diet?
    A. Meat
    B. Dairy
    C. Vegetables
    D. Nuts

35. What does the passage say is the idea behind the diet?
    A. That humans are genetically adapted to the diet of our Paleolithic forebears
    B. That it increases health
    C. That it supports weight loss
    D. That it consists of food that can be hunted or gathered

36. Which of the following does the passage suggest is true?
    A. No studies support the claim that the Paleolithic Diet promotes health
    B. Some studies support the claim that the Paleolithic Diet promotes health
    C. All studies support the claim that the Paleolithic Diet promotes health
    D. No studies have been done on whether the Paleolithic Diet promotes health

Questions 37-41 refer to the following medication directions:
    Directions: For the relief of headaches. Take one pill every 4 to 6 hours, not exceeding 4 in a 24-hour period. If stomach upset occurs, take with food. If pain persists more than 24 hours, contact a physician.

37. The medication should be taken:
    A. 6 times a day
    B. Every thirty minutes
    C. On an empty stomach
    D. To treat a headache

38. <u>Upset</u> means:
    A. Angry
    B. Annoyed
    C. Physical disorder
    D. Confusion

39. If someone follows the directions, what is the maximum number of pills he or she should have taken before he or she could first contact a physician?
    A. 2
    B. 3
    C. 4
    D. 6

40. <u>Persists</u> means
   A. Tries
   B. Continues
   C. Hurts
   D. Worsens

41. What is the maximum number of pills, including the first one, that could be taken in the 12 hours upon starting to use this medication?
   A. 2
   B. 3
   C. 4
   D. 5

Questions 42-47 refer to the following medication directions:

Tips for Eating Calcium Rich Foods
   - Include milk as a beverage at meals. Choose fat-free or low-fat milk.
   - If you usually drink whole milk, switch gradually to fat-free milk to lower saturated fat and calories. Try reduced fat (2%), then low-fat (1%), and finally fat-free (skim).
   - If you drink cappuccinos or lattes—ask for them with fat-free (skim) milk.
   - Add fat-free or low-fat milk instead of water to oatmeal and hot cereals
   - Use fat-free or low-fat milk when making condensed cream soups (such as cream of tomato).
   - Have fat-free or low-fat yogurt as a snack.
   - Make a dip for fruits or vegetables from yogurt.
   - Make fruit-yogurt smoothies in the blender.
   - For dessert, make chocolate or butterscotch pudding with fat-free or low-fat milk.
   - Top cut-up fruit with flavored yogurt for a quick dessert.
   - Top casseroles, soups, stews, or vegetables with shredded low-fat cheese.
   - Top a baked potato with fat-free or low-fat yogurt.

For those who choose not to consume milk products:
   - If you avoid milk because of lactose intolerance, the most reliable way to get the health benefits of milk is to choose lactose-free alternatives within the milk group, such as cheese, yogurt, or lactose-free milk, or to consume the enzyme lactase before consuming milk products.
   - Calcium choices for those who do not consume milk products include:
     o Calcium fortified juices, cereals, breads, soy beverages, or rice beverages
     o Canned fish (sardines, salmon with bones) soybeans and other soy products, some other dried beans, and some leafy greens.

42. According to the passage, how can you lower saturated fat and calories in your diet?
   A. Add fat-free milk to oatmeal instead of water
   B. Switch to fat-free milk
   C. Drink calcium-fortified juice
   D. Make yogurt dip

43. What device does the author use to organize the passage?
    A. Headings
    B. Captions
    C. Diagrams
    D. Labels

44. How much fat does reduced fat milk contain?
    A. 0 percent
    B. 1 percent
    C. 2 percent
    D. 3 percent

45. Which of the following is true about calcium rich foods?
    I. Canned salmon with bones contains calcium
    II. Cheese is a lactose-free food
    III. Condensed soup made with water is a calcium rich food
    A. I only
    B. I and II only
    C. II and III only
    D. III only

46. What information should the author include to help clarify information in the passage?
    A. The fat content of yogurt
    B. How much calcium is in fortified juice
    C. Which leafy greens contain calcium
    D. The definition of lactose intolerance

47. The style of this passage is most like that found in a(n):
    A. Tourist guidebook
    B. Teen magazine
    C. Encyclopedia
    D. Health textbook

Section 2. Vocabulary and General Knowledge	Number of Questions: **50**
	Time Limit: **50 Minutes**

1. What is the best definition for the word *latent*?
    A. Thorough
    B. Dormant
    C. Current
    D. Obvious

2. What is the meaning of the word *precipitous*?
    A. Cautious
    B. Languid
    C. Subtle
    D. Abrupt

3. What is the best definition of the word *recur*?
    A. Redo
    B. Recreate
    C. Return
    D. Revolve

4. What is the meaning of the word *diffuse*?
    A. Disseminate
    B. Compress
    C. Distinct
    D. Widen

5. What is the meaning of the word *anterior*?
    A. Previous
    B. Front
    C. Crucial
    D. Final

6. What is the meaning of the word *insidious*?
    A. Reliable
    B. Limited
    C. Rapid
    D. Subtle

7. What is the best definition for the word *comply*?
    A. Follow
    B. Affect
    C. Depend
    D. Decline

8. Select the meaning of the underlined word in this sentence:
Despite the leadership problems that plagued the corporation, the CEO was quick to <u>assert</u> his authority to ensure that business continued as usual.
  A. Maintain
  B. Prevent
  C. Censure
  D. Accept

9. What is the meaning of the word *occlude*?
  A. Release
  B. Invade
  C. Prevent
  D. Direct

10. Select the meaning of the underlined word in this sentence:
Having spent hours preparing her research, Eirinn felt that her colleague's hasty rejection of her presentation was <u>untoward</u> and merited a formal complaint.
  A. Inappropriate
  B. Delicate
  C. Friendly
  D. Eager

11. What is the best definition for the word *superficial*?
  A. Surface
  B. Backward
  C. Awkward
  D. Intense

12. What is the best definition for the word *inverted*?
  A. Credible
  B. Benign
  C. Forward
  D. Reversed

13. What is the meaning of the word *void*?
  A. Emit
  B. Determine
  C. Confirm
  D. Prevent

14. Select the meaning of the underlined word in this sentence:
Fearful that the fever might have an <u>adverse</u> effect, Catriona called the doctor for an emergency appointment.
  A. Preventive
  B. Auspicious
  C. Negative
  D. Reckless

15. What is the meaning of the word *contingent*?
    A. Dependent
    B. Protective
    C. Definite
    D. Intended

16. Select the meaning of the underlined word in this sentence:
Philippa was upset about the doctor's unwillingness to release her from the hospital for another week, so she demanded that he explain his <u>rationale</u> to her.
    A. Description
    B. Justification
    C. Persistence
    D. Ambiguity

17. What is the best definition for the word *patent*?
    A. Inconspicuous
    B. Privileged
    C. Careless
    D. Unconcealed

18. What is the best definition for the word *labile*?
    A. External
    B. Meticulous
    C. Fluctuating
    D. Integral

19. What is the best definition for the word *impending*?
    A. Demanding
    B. Approaching
    C. Perilous
    D. Producing

20. What is the meaning of the word *exacerbate*?
    A. Aggravate
    B. Exaggerate
    C. Outrage
    D. Alleviate

21. What is the meaning of the word *lethargic*?
    A. Calm
    B. Sluggish
    C. Conscious
    D. Elaborate

22. Select the meaning of the underlined word in this sentence:
Niamh noticed the crumbs on her young son's face and wondered that he could tell such an <u>overt</u> lie about not eating any cookies.
    A. Unnecessary
    B. Tangible
    C. Energetic
    D. Obvious

23. What is the best definition for the word *discrete*?
    A. Standard
    B. Subtle
    C. Normal
    D. Separate

24. What is the best definition for the word *adsorb*?
    A. Divide
    B. Process
    C. Accumulate
    D. Contain

25. What is the best definition for the word *compensatory*?
    A. Corrupted
    B. Offsetting
    C. Varying
    D. Contradictory

26. What is the meaning of the word *incompatible*?
    A. Conflicting
    B. Subsequent
    C. Relevant
    D. Suitable

27. What is the best definition for the word *lateral*?
    A. Positive
    B. Central
    C. Sideward
    D. Serious

28. What is the meaning of the word *distended*?
    A. Embellished
    B. Abridged
    C. Tightened
    D. Bulging

29. What is the meaning of the word *exiguous*?
    A. Superfluous
    B. Defective
    C. Inadequate
    D. Eager

30. What is the meaning of the word *untenable*?
    A. Logical
    B. Groundless
    C. Opaque
    D. Analogous

31. What is the best definition for the word *placate*?
    A. Authorize
    B. Incite
    C. Clarify
    D. Comfort

32. What is the best definition for the word *inure*?
    A. Toughen
    B. Pretend
    C. Anticipate
    D. Forget

33. What is the best definition for the word *clement*?
    A. Difficult
    B. Angry
    C. Favorable
    D. Righteous

34. What is the meaning of the word *malign*?
    A. Harm
    B. Submit
    C. Improve
    D. Conceive

35. What is the best definition for the word *synergy*?
    A. Delay
    B. Harmony
    C. Distress
    D. Hindrance

36. What is the best definition for the word *recede*?
    A. Increase
    B. Dilate
    C. Present
    D. Retreat

37. What is the best definition for the word *inflame*?
    A. Worsen
    B. Ignite
    C. Lull
    D. Endanger

38. What is the meaning of the word *detriment*?
    A. Drawback
    B. Retribution
    C. Excitement
    D. Indulgence

39. What is the meaning of the word *turgid*?
    A. Intricate
    B. Murky
    C. Inflated
    D. Acceptable

40. What is the meaning of the word *paucity*?
    A. Hunger
    B. Affluence
    C. Lack
    D. Insistence

41. What is the best definition for the word *proscribe*?
    A. Belittle
    B. Increase
    C. Praise
    D. Forbid

42. What is the meaning of the word *austere*?
    A. Calm
    B. Stark
    C. Dependable
    D. Greedy

43. What is the best definition for the word *delineate*?
    A. Open
    B. Confuse
    C. Brag
    D. Detail

44. What is the best definition for the word *expedient*?
    A. Grateful
    B. Practical
    C. Unprofitable
    D. Substitute

45. What is the meaning of the word *facilitate*?
    A. recast
    B. smooth
    C. thwart
    D. decide

46. What is the meaning of the word *restive*?
    A. Frightened
    B. Hostile
    C. Tense
    D. Apathetic

47. What is the best definition for the word *recourse*?
    A. Ambush
    B. Obligation
    C. Option
    D. Proposal

48. What is the best definition for the word *impetus*?
    A. Motivation
    B. Diversion
    C. Authority
    D. Prevention

49. What is the best definition for the word *salient*?
    A. Acceptable
    B. Ordinary
    C. Peripheral
    D. Important

50. What is the meaning of the word *laconic*?
    A. Slow
    B. Incomplete
    C. Brief
    D. Tidy

Section 3. Grammar

Number of Questions: **50**
Time Limit: **50 Minutes**

1. Select the word that makes this sentence grammatically correct:
Writing, doing yoga, and _____ were her favorite activities.
   A. playing volleyball
   B. doing volleyball
   C. making volleyball
   D. volleyballing

2. Select the word that makes this sentence grammatically correct:
Every kid in the neighborhood has _____ own bicycle.
   A. its
   B. their
   C. our
   D. her

3. Select the word that makes this sentence grammatically correct:
Maria thinks it is unfair that she has to _____ with her younger brother's whining all the time.
   A. put up
   B. put down
   C. put in
   D. put off

4. Select the word that makes this sentence grammatically correct:
Enrique will _____ harder as the date of the test draws nearer.
   A. studying
   B. have studied
   C. studyed
   D. study

5. Select the word that makes this sentence grammatically correct:
Suzanna replied _____ to her sister's plea to help her with her finances.
   A. sympathelly
   B. sympathetically
   C. sympathetilly
   D. sympathetic

6. Select the word that makes this sentence grammatically correct:
A team of scientists _____ studying a new species of frog never found before.
   A. is
   B. are
   C. were
   D. have

7. Select the word that makes this sentence grammatically correct:
Everyone we invited to the party _____, so it was a huge success!
   A. shown up
   B. showed up
   C. showed upped
   D. shows up

8. Which word is not spelled correctly in the context of the following sentence?
Buying prescents for others is not the most authentic way to develop new friendships.
   A. buying
   B. prescents
   C. authentic
   D. friendships

9. Which word is not spelled correctly in the context of the following sentence?
Raymond feels children misbehave too much, that parents have lost their athourity, and that they need to emphasize discipline more.
   A. misbehave
   B. emphasize
   C. discipline
   D. athourity

10. Select the word that makes this sentence grammatically correct:
Each received _____ trophy to take home.
   A. it's
   B. her
   C. their
   D. our

11. Select the word that makes this sentence grammatically correct:
Eli _____ insisted that it wasn't his fault.
   A. tearfully
   B. tearilly
   C. with tears
   D. teary

12. Select the word that makes this sentence grammatically correct:
Margaret _____ the committee into thinking the project was all her work.
   A. missled
   B. misled
   C. mislead
   D. mislled

13. Select the word that makes this sentence grammatically correct:
Tomorrow, Atticus will _____ cupcakes to school.
   A. brought
   B. had brought
   C. bring
   D. broughten

14. Select the word that makes this sentence grammatically correct:
Each participant in the course on being a good father received _____ signed copy of the teacher's book.
    A. their
    B. our
    C. his
    D. ones

15. Select the word that makes this sentence grammatically correct:
Several of the runners _____ not to complete the race; they met the rest of us by the finish line.
    A. decide
    B. decided
    C. decides
    D. were deciding

16. Select the word that makes this sentence grammatically correct:
Stephanie writes _____.
    A. good
    B. well
    C. clear
    D. more

17. Which word is not spelled correctly in the context of the following sentence?
Judy's neighbor was friends with her neice and invited her on the holiday sleigh ride.
    A. Neighbor
    B. Friends
    C. Neice
    D. Sleigh

18. Which word is not spelled correctly in the context of the following sentence?
Oscar was truly sad to be enforcing the hateful judgement.
    A. truly
    B. enforcing
    C. hateful
    D. judgement

19. Select the word or phrase that makes the following sentence grammatically correct.
Everyone who visits the fine art museum _____ to see the new Manet exhibit.
    A. should
    B. needs
    C. have
    D. must

20. Select the word or phrase that makes the following sentence grammatically correct.
Their experience at the opera, viewing the company's production of Turandot, was so bad that _____ have yet returned.
    A. he and she
    B. we
    C. him and her
    D. him and I

21. Select the word or phrase that makes the following sentence grammatically correct.
After hearing about everyone's positive experience at the party, Desmond realized that he _____.
   A. should have went
   B. should have gone
   C. should go
   D. should have been

22. Select the word or phrase that makes the following sentence grammatically correct.
Loman made a quick telephone call to the person _____ was responsible for organizing the event.
   A. that
   B. which
   C. who
   D. this

23. Select the word or phrase that makes the following sentence grammatically correct.
Nessa returned the lost cat to the Millers after seeing the sign and realizing that the cat was _____.
   A. hers
   B. his
   C. ours
   D. theirs

24. Select the word or phrase that makes the following sentence grammatically correct.
See to it that Derek or Una _____ the box of clothing that is to be donated to the church rummage sale.
   A. are collecting
   B. collects
   C. collect
   D. would collect

25. Select the word or phrase that makes the following sentence grammatically correct.
Neither Jane nor _____ knows at what time the surprise party for Richard is supposed to begin.
   A. she
   B. him
   C. me
   D. they

26. Select the word or phrase that makes the following sentence grammatically correct.
Ieva pointed a quivering finger at the butler and exclaimed, "It was _____! He stole the pearls from my room."
   A. him
   B. his
   C. himself
   D. he

27. Select the word or phrase that makes the following sentence grammatically correct.
The grand prize of $10,000 will be given to _____ arrives at the finish line first.
   A. who
   B. whom
   C. whoever
   D. whomever

3 HESI Admission Assessment Practice Tests

28. Select the word or phrase that makes the following sentence grammatically correct.
Angus knew his mobile phone was gone for good when he realized that he had forgotten to take it _____ the roof of the car before he started driving.
    A. off
    B. off of
    C. off from
    D. away from

29. Select the word or phrase that makes the following sentence grammatically correct.
The committee _____ in disagreement about the decorations for the upcoming event.
    A. is
    B. were
    C. was
    D. would be

30. Select the word or phrase that makes the following sentence grammatically correct.
About three o'clock in the afternoon, a parched Veronika realized that she had not _____ any water all day.
    A. drank
    B. drunk
    C. drink
    D. drunken

31. Select the word or phrase that makes the following sentence grammatically correct.
The priest quoted I Corinthians 2.9: "What no eye has _____, what no ear has heard, and what no human mind has conceived…"
    A. saw
    B. see
    C. seeing
    D. seen

32. Select the word or phrase that makes the following sentence grammatically correct.
When the ice-cream man arrives later today, the children _____.
    A. were excited
    B. would be excited
    C. will be excited
    D. would have been excited

33. Select the word or phrase that makes the following sentence grammatically correct.
Once I complete this final pose, I _____ yoga for two full hours.
    A. will have been doing
    B. will do
    C. will be doing
    D. would be doing

34. Select the word or phrase that makes the following sentence grammatically correct.
Effie contacted a travel agent to help her find the vacation plan _____ offered her the best options.
    A. that
    B. than
    C. which
    D. who

3 HESI Admission Assessment Practice Tests   119

35. Select the word or phrase that makes the following sentence grammatically correct.
Aidan performed the solo _____, far worse than anyone had expected.
  A. real bad
  B. real badly
  C. really bad
  D. really badly

36. Select the word or phrase that makes the following sentence grammatically correct.
Grant demanded of his teenage son, "_____?"
  A. Where did you go to
  B. Where did you go from
  C. Where did you go at
  D. Where did you go

37. Select the word or phrase that makes the following sentence grammatically correct.
I should _____ attended the concert, since everyone mentioned how fun it was.
  A. of
  B. be
  C. have
  D. has

38. Select the punctuation that makes the following sentence grammatically correct.
When Finn called his mother he did not tell her about all of his plans.
  A. mother, he
  B. Finn, called
  C. not, tell
  D. when, Finn

39. Select the word or phrase that makes the following sentence grammatically correct.
Professor Howard had thirty-five students in the class, and she stayed up late grading all the _____ papers.
  A. student's
  B. students
  C. students's
  D. students'

40. Select the word or phrase that makes the following sentence grammatically correct.
The kindergarten teacher praised Kama after she did _____ on the assignment.
  A. good
  B. great
  C. worse
  D. well

41. Select the punctuation that makes the following sentence grammatically correct.
Olaf planned to see the movie but he could not go after he caught the flu.
  A. but, he
  B. movie, he
  C. movie, but
  D. but; he

42. Select the word or phrase that makes the following sentence grammatically correct.
Maura knocked on the door of _____ dorm room.
    A. Melissa and Caroline's
    B. Melissa's and Caroline
    C. Melissa's and Caroline's
    D. Melissa and Caroline

43. Select the expression that uses the correct punctuation to complete the following sentence.
Doctor Marshall has had his medical license since the early _____.
    A. 1980's
    B. 1980s'
    C. 1980s
    D. '1980s

44. Select the word or phrase that makes the following sentence grammatically correct.
Jean intended to hold the picnic on Saturday, _____ the sudden deluge forced her to reschedule it.
    A. and
    B. however
    C. but
    D. or

45. Select the word or phrase that makes the following sentence grammatically correct.
The professor announced to the class, "To prevent the temptation for cheating, I will collect your study notes _____ the exam."
    A. during
    B. before
    C. upon
    D. after

46. Select the combination of words that makes the following sentence grammatically correct.
I want to _____ a change in the program, so I will have to present a solution that will have a strong _____ on the board.
    A. affect, affect
    B. affect, effect
    C. effect, effect
    D. effect, affect

47. Select the combination of words that makes the following sentence grammatically correct.
Due to company policy, Eleanora could not _____ any gifts _____ from other company employees, and only on her birthday.
    A. accept, except
    B. accept, accept
    C. except, accept
    D. except, except

48. Select the combination of words that makes the following sentence grammatically correct.
To _____ that you are properly covered, be sure to _____ your home against fire.
    A. ensure, ensure
    B. insure, insure
    C. insure, ensure
    D. ensure, insure

49. Disney films often use the same voice actors; _____, Sterling Holloway was the voice for Winnie the Pooh, the stork in Dumbo, the snake Kaa in Jungle Book, and the Cheshire Cat in Alice in Wonderland.
    A. but
    B. for instance
    C. thus
    D. so

50. Choose the word or words that best fill the blank.
Many similarities exist between the film Star Wars IV: A New Hope and a Japanese film called The Hidden Fortress; _____ , Star Wars director George Lucas openly acknowledges the film as a significant influence.
    A. however
    B. or
    C. in fact
    D. yet

Section 3. Mathematics

Number of Questions: **50**	
Time Limit: **50 Minutes**	

1. 25% of 400 =
   A. 100
   B. 200
   C. 800
   D. 10,000

2. What is the reciprocal of 6?
   A. ½
   B. 1/3
   C. 1/6
   D. 1/12

3. A roast was cooked at 325 °F in the oven for 4 hours. The internal temperature rose from 32 °F to 145 °F. What was the average rise in temperature per hour?
   A. 20.2 °F/hr
   B. 28.25°F/hr
   C. 32.03°F/hr
   D. 37°F/hr

4. Your supervisor instructs you to purchase 240 pens and 6 staplers for the nurse's station. Pens are purchase in sets of 6 for $2.35 per pack. Staplers are sold in sets of 2 for 12.95. How much will purchasing these products cost?
   A. $132.85
   B. $145.75
   C. $162.90
   D. $225.05

5. Which of the following percentages is equal to 0.45?
   A. 0.045%
   B. 0.45%
   C. 4.5%
   D. 45%

6. A vitamin's expiration date has passed. It was suppose to contain 500 mg of Calcium, but it has lost 325 mg of Calcium. How many mg of Calcium is left?
   A. 135 mg
   B. 175 mg
   C. 185 mg
   D. 200 mg

7. You have orders to give a patient 20 mg of a certain medication. The medication is stored 4 mg per 5-mL dose. How many milliliters will need to be given?
   A. 15 mL
   B. 20 mL
   C. 25 mL
   D. 30 mL

8. In the number 743.25 which digit represents the tenths space?
   A. 2
   B. 3
   C. 4
   D. 5

9. Which of these percentages equals 1.25?
   A. 0.125%
   B. 12.5%
   C. 125%
   D. 1250%

10. If the average person drinks 8, (8oz) glasses of water per day, a person who drinks 12.8 oz of water after a morning exercise session has consumed what fraction of the daily average?
   A. 1/3
   B. 1/5
   C. 1/7
   D. 1/9

11. 33% of 300 =
   A. 3
   B. 9
   C. 33
   D. 99

12. You need 4/5 cups of water for a recipe. You accidentally put 1/3 cups into the mixing bowl with the dry ingredients. How much more water in cups do you need to add?
   A. 1/3 cups
   B. 2/3 cups
   C. 1/15 cups
   D. 7/15 cups

13. ¾ - ½ =
   A. ¼
   B. 1/3
   C. ½
   D. 2/3

14. In your class there are 48 students, 32 students are female. Approximately what percentage is male?
   A. 25%
   B. 33%
   C. 45%
   D. 66%

15. Fried's rule for computing an infant's dose of medication is:

Child's age in months

infant's dose = X adult dose

150

If the adult dose of medication is 15 mg, how much should be given to a 2 year-old child?

A. 1.2

B. 2.4

C. 3.6

D. 4.8

16. 7 ½ - 5 3/8 =

A. 1 ½

B. 1 2/3

C. 2 1/8

D. 3 ¼

17. 35 is 20% of what number?

A. 175

B. 186

C. 190

D. 220

18. 6 x 0 x 5

A. 30

B. 11

C. 25

D. 0

19. 7.95 ÷ 1.5

A. 2.4

B. 5.3

C. 6.2

D. 7.3

20. 7/10 equals:

A. .007

B. .07

C. .7

D. 1.7

21. 4/8 equals:

A. 0.005

B. 0.05

C. 0.5

D. 1.5

22. −32 + 7 equals:

A. −25

B. 25

C. −26

D. 26

23. 41% equals:
   A. 4.1
   B. .41
   C. .041
   D. .0041

24. 248 + 311
   A. 557
   B. 559
   C. 659
   D. 667

25. 13,980 + 7,031
   A. 20,010
   B. 20.911
   C. 21,011
   D. 21,911

26. 8,537 - 6,316
   A. 1,221
   B. 2,221
   C. 2,243
   D. 2,841

27. 643 x 72
   A. 44,096
   B. 44,186
   C. 46,296
   D. 45,576

28. $63\overline{)18144}$
   A. 256
   B. 258
   C. 286
   D. 288

29. 3.5 + 10.3 + 0.63
   A. 11.28
   B. 13.58
   C. 14.43
   D. 20.10

30. 0.19 x 0.23
   A. .3470
   B. .4370
   C. .0347
   D. .0437

31. $\dfrac{0.3}{0.08}$ is equal to
    A. .0375
    B. .375
    C. 3.75
    D. 37.5

32. Which numeral is in the thousandths place in .5643?
    A. 5
    B. 6
    C. 4
    D. 3

33. 0.43 - 0.17
    A. .26
    B. 2.6
    C. .36
    D. 3.6

34. Round off to the nearest hundredth .3489
    A. .33
    B. .349
    C. .348
    D. .35

35. $2\frac{1}{2} + 3 + \frac{1}{7}$
    A. 5 9/14
    B. 6 1/2
    C. 5 5/14
    D. 6 5/7

36. $3\frac{1}{9} - 1\frac{1}{4} =$
    A. $1\frac{5}{6}$
    B. $1\frac{31}{36}$
    C. $2\frac{5}{36}$
    D. $2\frac{31}{36}$

37. $3\frac{1}{8} \, x \, 6\frac{1}{3} \, x \, 2\frac{2}{5}$
    A. $47\frac{1}{2}$
    B. $36\frac{7}{8}$
    C. $40\frac{3}{8}$
    D. $42\frac{4}{5}$

38. $\frac{1}{8} \div \frac{4}{5}$

    A. $\frac{5}{32}$

    B. $\frac{1}{10}$

    C. $\frac{2}{5}$

    D. $\frac{3}{8}$

39. Find N for the following:

$$\frac{n}{5} = \frac{12}{20}$$

    A. 2

    B. 3

    C. 4

    D. 5

40. Reduce $\frac{17}{102}$ to lowest terms.

    A. $\frac{1}{4}$

    B. $\frac{5}{6}$

    C. $\frac{1}{6}$

    D. $\frac{3}{4}$

41. Express 99/14 as a mixed fraction.

    A. $7\frac{1}{14}$

    B. $7\frac{3}{14}$

    C. $7\frac{11}{14}$

    D. $7\frac{5}{14}$

42. 3 is what percent of 50?

    A. 3%

    B. 4%

    C. 5%

    D. 6%

43. Three fifths of sixty equals:

    A. 30

    B. 32

    C. 36

    D. 40

44. 0.5% of 40=

    A. .2

    B. .8

    C. 2.0

    D. 8.0

45. Ratio of 2 to 10 = (?)%
    A. 2
    B. 3
    C. 5
    D. 20

46. $\frac{3}{5}$ as a percentage
    A. 40%
    B. 4%
    C. 60%
    D. 6%

47. 15% as a reduced common fraction
    A. $\frac{3}{20}$
    B. $\frac{15}{100}$
    C. $\frac{5}{20}$
    D. $\frac{20}{3}$

48. $1\frac{1}{4}$% of (?) = 1.5
    A. 80
    B. 120
    C. 140
    D. 150

49. 8 is 25% of x
    A. 16
    B. 24
    C. 32
    D. 40

50. 40% of x=18
    A. 36
    B. 360
    C. 45
    D. 450

Section 5. Biology

| Number of Questions: **25** |
| Time Limit: **25 Minutes** |

1. Which of the following sentences is true?
    A. All organisms begin life as a single cell
    B. All organisms begin life as multi-cellular
    C. Some organisms begin life as a single cell and others as multi-cellular
    D. None of the above

2. Which of the following is the best definition for metabolism?
    A. The process by which organisms lose weight
    B. The process by which organisms use energy
    C. The process by which organisms return to homeostasis
    D. The process by which organisms leave homeostasis

3. Which of the following is not true for all cells?
    A. Cells are the basic structures of any organism
    B. Cells can only reproduce from existing cells
    C. Cells are the smallest unit of any life form that carries the information needed for all life processes
    D. All cells are also called eukaryotes

4. What are the two types of cellular transport?
    A. Passive and diffusion
    B. Diffusion and active
    C. Active and passive
    D. Kinetic and active

5. What does aerobic mean?
    A. In the presence of oxygen
    B. Calorie-burning
    C. Heated
    D. Anabolic

6. When both parents give offspring the same allele, the offspring is _____ for that trait.
    A. Heterozygous
    B. Homozygous
    C. Recessive
    D. Dominant

7. Genetics is the study of:
    A. Anatomy
    B. Physiology
    C. Heredity
    D. Science

8. Scientists suggest that _____ has occurred through a process called _____.
   A. evolution... differentiation
   B. evolution... natural selection
   C. natural selection... homeostasis
   D. homeostasis... reproduction

9. Which of the following correctly lists the cellular hierarchy from the simplest to the most complex structure?
   A. tissue, cell, organ, organ system, organism
   B. organism, organ system, organ, tissue, cell
   C. organ system, organism, organ, tissue, cell
   D. cell, tissue, organ, organ system, organism

10. If a cell is placed in a hypertonic solution, what will happen to the cell?
    A. It will swell
    B. It will shrink
    C. It will stay the same
    D. It does not affect the cell

11. What is the longest phase of the cell cycle?
    A. mitosis
    B. cytokinesis
    C. interphase
    D. metaphase

Use the following Punnett Square to answer questions 12 and 13:
   B = alleles for brown eyes; g = alleles for green eyes

	B	g
B	BB	Bg
g	Bg	gg

12. Which word describes the allele for green eyes?
    A. dominant
    B. recessive
    C. homozygous
    D. heterozygous

13. What is the possibility that the offspring produced will have brown eyes?
    A. 25%
    B. 50%
    C. 75%
    D. 100%

14. Which of the following correctly describes the trait Ll, if "L" represents tallness and "l" represents shortness?
    A. heterozygous genotype and tall phenotype
    B. heterozygous phenotype and tall genotype
    C. homozygous genotype and short phenotype
    D. homozygous phenotype and short genotype

15. Which of the following is an example of a non-communicable disease?
    A. influenza
    B. tuberculosis
    C. arthritis
    D. measles

16. All living organisms on Earth utilize:
    A. Oxygen
    B. Light
    C. Sexual reproduction
    D. A triplet genetic code

17. Which of the following is not a nitrogenous base found in DNA?
    A. Thymine
    B. Uracil
    C. Guanine
    D. Adenine

18. Which of the following is true?
    A. The basic formula for a carbohydrate is $(CH_2O)_N$
    B. Water bonds well with nonpolar substances
    C. Enzymes are an example of secondary proteins
    D. An exergonic reaction is one that uses up energy

19. Which cell structure is responsible for modifying substances and distributing them to their proper place in the cell?
    A. Endoplasmic reticulum
    B. Ribosome
    C. Golgi apparatus
    D. Lysosome

20. Prokaryotes do not contain:
    A. cell membrane
    B. cell wall
    C. nucleus
    D. ribosomes

21. Which stage of mitosis is occurring when the centromeres are lining up in the middle of the cell and preparing for division?
    A. Metaphase
    B. Anaphase
    C. Prophase
    D. Telophase

22. During the S phase in the Interphase stage of mitosis, what event is occurring?
    A. Resting before the next cell division
    B. Rapid DNA replication
    C. Cytokinesis
    D. Construction of microtubules which will eventually form the cytoskeleton

23. Which of the following is true of meiosis?
    A. Two identical daughter cells are formed
    B. It is used to replicate body cells
    C. Four diploid cells are formed during Meiosis II
    D. Gametes are haploid cells

24. Which of the following statements about the Krebs cycle is true?
    A. It occurs only once per glucose molecule
    B. It is an anaerobic process
    C. It takes place in the cytoplasm
    D. It starts with the conversion of one pyruvate molecule into 2 acetyl-CoA molecules

25. How is the most amount of energy released from ATP?
    A. When the entire molecule of ATP has been broken apart
    B. When ADP binds to another phosphate group to form ATP
    C. When one phosphate group breaks off ATP to form ADP and free phosphate
    D. Each time an additional phosphate group bonds with adenosine, forming ADP and then ATP

Section 6. Chemistry

| Number of Questions: 25 |
| Time Limit: 25 Minutes |

1. Which of the following is true?
   A. Mass and weight are the same thing
   B. Mass is the quantity of matter an object has
   C. Mass equals twice the weight of an object
   D. Mass equals half the weight of an object

2. Which of the following is not a state of matter?
   A. Gas
   B. Liquid
   C. Lattice
   D. Solid

3. What is the name for substances that cannot be broken down into simpler types of matter?
   A. Electron
   B. Molecules
   C. Nuclei
   D. Elements

4. What are the two types of measurement important in science?
   A. quantitative and numerical
   B. qualitative and descriptive
   C. numerical and scientific
   D. quantitative and qualitative

5. What is the typical way a solid would turn to a liquid and then to a gas?
   A. Vaporization then melting
   B. Melting then freezing
   C. Vaporization then freezing
   D. Melting then vaporization

6. An atom with an electrical charge is called a(n):
   A. Electron
   B. Ion
   C. Molecule
   D. Enzyme

7. When atoms of one element are combined with atoms of another element, the result is a(n) _____ of a compound.
   A. Electron
   B. Ion
   C. Molecule
   D. Enzyme

8. What is freezing point?
   A. The point at which a liquid changes to a solid
   B. The point at which a gas changes to a liquid
   C. The point at which a gas changes to a solid
   D. The point at which a liquid changes to a gas

9. The rate of a chemical reaction depends on all of the following except:
   A. temperature
   B. surface area
   C. presence of catalysts
   D. amount of mass lost

10. Which of the answer choices provided best defines the following statement:
For a given mass and constant temperature, an inverse relationship exists between the volume and pressure of a gas?
   A. Ideal Gas Law
   B. Boyle's Law
   C. Charles' Law
   D. Stefan-Boltzmann Law

11. Which of the following is exchanged between two or more atoms that undergo ionic bonding?
   A. neutrons
   B. transitory electrons
   C. valence electrons
   D. electrical charges

12. Which of the following statements is *not* true of most metals?
   A. They are good conductors of heat
   B. They are gases at room temperature
   C. They are ductile
   D. They make up the majority of elements on the periodic table

13. What is most likely the pH of a solution containing many hydroxide ions (OH^-) and few hydrogen ions (H^+)?
   A. 2
   B. 6
   C. 7
   D. 9

14. Which of the following cannot be found on the periodic table?
   A. bromine
   B. magnesium oxide
   C. phosphorous
   D. chlorine

15. Nora makes soup by adding some spices to a pot of boiling water and stirring the spices until completely dissolved. Next, she adds several chopped vegetables. What is the solute in her mixture?
   A. water
   B. vegetables
   C. spices
   D. heat

3 HESI Admission Assessment Practice Tests

16. What law describes the electric force between two charged particles?
     A. Ohm's law
     B. Coulomb's law
     C. The Doppler effect
     D. Kirchhoff's current law

17. What process transfers thermal energy through matter directly from particle to particle?
     A. convection
     B. radiation
     C. conduction
     D. insulation

18. Which state of matter contains the least amount of kinetic energy?
     A. solid
     B. liquid
     C. gas
     D. plasma

19. Which of the following is a vector quantity?
     A. Distance
     B. Speed
     C. Velocity
     D. Time

20. As you move from left to right across the periodic table, which of the following is true?
     A. Atomic radius increases
     B. Electronegativity increases
     C. Ionization energy decreases
     D. Electron affinity decreases

21. What is the correct molecular formula for aluminum hydroxide?
     A. $Al(OH)_3$
     B. $AlOH_3$
     C. Al_3OH
     D. AlO_3H

22. According to Boyle's law:
     A. $PV = nRT$
     B. temperature and volume are directly related
     C. the volume of a gas is inversely related to the number of moles in that gas
     D. pressure and volume of a gas are inversely related

23. What type of substance has some properties of a metal, but is made up of a mixture of different elements?
     A. Metals
     B. Nonmetals
     C. Alloy
     D. Network solids

24. The process of sublimation occurs when a _____ changes into a _____.
   A. solid, gas
   B. liquid, gas
   C. gas, solid
   D. liquid, solid

25. Decreasing a liquid's pH from 5 to 4 will increase the hydrogen ion concentration by a factor of:
   A. 10
   B. 100
   C. 1,000
   D. 10,000

Section 7. Anatomy and Physiology	Number of Questions: 25
	Time Limit: **25 Minutes**

1. Which hormone is *not* secreted by a gland in the brain?
   A. Human chorionic gonadotropin (HCG)
   B. Gonadotropin releasing hormone (GnRH)
   C. Luteinizing hormone (LH)
   D. Follicle stimulating hormone (FSH)

2. How many basic tissue types does a human have?
   A. 4
   B. 6
   C. 12
   D. 23

3. Which of the following is not a type of muscle tissue?
   A. Skeletal
   B. Smooth
   C. Cardiac
   D. Adipose

4. Which of the following organ systems has the purpose of producing movement through contraction?
   A. Skeletal
   B. Muscular
   C. Cardiovascular
   D. Respiratory

5. Which of the following terms means toward the front of the body?
   A. Superior
   B. Anterior
   C. Inferior
   D. Posterior

6. The brain is part of the:
   A. Integumentary system
   B. Nervous system
   C. Endocrine system
   D. Respiratory system

7. Which of the following is the name for the study of the structure and shape of the human body?
   A. Physiology
   B. Anatomy
   C. Biology
   D. Genetics

8. Which of the following is the name for the study of how parts of the body function?
   A. Physiology
   B. Anatomy
   C. Biology
   D. Genetics

9. Which of the below is the best definition for the term circulation?
   A. The transport of oxygen and other nutrients to the tissues via the cardiovascular system
   B. The force exerted by blood against a unit area of the blood vessel walls
   C. The branching air passageways inside the lungs
   D. The process of breathing in

10. Which of the following is not a type of connective tissue?
    A. smooth
    B. cartilage
    C. adipose tissue
    D. blood tissue

11. How many organ systems are there in the human body?
    A. 4
    B. 7
    C. 11
    D. 13

12. Which organ system includes the spleen?
    A. Endocrine
    B. Lymphatic
    C. Respiratory
    D. Digestive

13. Which of the following terms means close to the trunk of the body?
    A. Superficial
    B. Sagittal
    C. Proximal
    D. Distal

14. Which of the following does the integumentary system, the skin, NOT do?
    A. Protect internal tissues from injury
    B. Waterproofs the body
    C. Helps regulate body temperature
    D. Return fluid to the blood vessels

15. What does the term optic refer to?
    A. The eye or vision
    B. The ear or hearing
    C. The mouth or tasting
    D. The nose or smelling

16. What are groups of cells that perform the same function called?
    A. tissues
    B. plastids
    C. organs
    D. molecules

17. When does the nuclear division of somatic cells take place during cellular reproduction?
    A. meiosis
    B. cytokinesis
    C. interphase
    D. mitosis

18. Which group of major parts and organs make up the immune system?
    A. lymphatic system, spleen, tonsils, thymus, and bone marrow
    B. brain, spinal cord, and nerve cells
    C. heart, veins, arteries, and capillaries
    D. nose, trachea, bronchial tubes, lungs, alveolus, and diaphragm

19. What is the role of ribosomes?
    A. make proteins
    B. waste removal
    C. transport
    D. storage

20. Which of the following is an example of a tissue?
    A. cortical bone
    B. liver
    C. mammal
    D. hamstring

21. The adrenal glands are part of the
    A. immune system
    B. endocrine system
    C. emphatic system
    D. respiratory system

22. Hemoglobin transports oxygen from the lungs to the rest of the body, making oxygen available for cell use. What is hemoglobin?
    A. an enzyme
    B. a protein
    C. a lipid
    D. an acid

23. Which of the following statements describes the function of smooth muscle tissue?
    A. It contracts to force air into and out of the lungs
    B. It contracts to force air into and out of the stomach
    C. It contracts to support the spinal column
    D. It contracts to assist the stomach in the mechanical breakdown of food

24. Which of the following is not a product of respiration?
    A. carbon dioxide
    B. water
    C. glucose
    D. ATP

25. Of the following, the blood vessel containing the least-oxygenated blood is:
    A. The aorta
    B. The vena cava
    C. The pulmonary artery
    D. The capillaries

AnswerExplanations

ReadingComprehension Answer Key and Explanations

1. C: Sentence reads, "Your brain <u>filters</u> [your nose] out," which means your brain ignores it.

2. B: Only choice B reflects the meaning of the term "retina," which is a part of the eye's anatomy.

3. B: The final sentence reads, "Your brain works hard to make the world look continuous." It follows that visual perception is an active process, not a passive one, making choice B the best answer.

4. A: If the reader follows the instructions given in the paragraph, the O and X in the middle of the passage can be used to demonstrate the blind spot in the visual field. Choice A is the best answer.

5. B: The passage explains the way that visual perception works. Choice B is the best answer.

6. D: Much of the information in the passage is provided to show examples of how the brain fills in gaps in the visual field. Choice D is the best answer.

7. A: The author of the passage mentions the nose to demonstrate how the brain filters information out of the visual field. Choice A is the best answer.

8. B: Choice B can be inferred from the second paragraph. The paragraph states that the brain filters out information, which means that the brain does not perceive all activity in the visual field.

9. D: Of the given options, only choice D can be inferred from the passage. The passage reads that parents should "try not to <u>feed into</u> oppositional behavior by reacting emotionally," which implies that reacting emotionally to defiant behavior can worsen it.

10. B: Choice B, "ODD is a complex condition" is the best answer out of the four given. It is the only choice that can be inferred from the passage as a whole.

11. A: Choice A is the best choice. Oppositional means uncooperative.

12. B: Choice B is the best interpretation of paragraph one. The passage states that many people exhibit ODD symptoms from time to time.

13. C: Choice C is the best choice. <u>Feed into</u> in this sentence means to encourage oppositional behavior.

14. C: Someone with <u>low frustration tolerance</u> has a difficult time tolerating or dealing with frustration. Choice C is the best answer.

15. C: This passage is meant to inform the reader about ODD. Choice C is the best choice.

16. C: While some of these answer choices may contribute to ODD, the passage mentions only choice C, severe or unpredictable punishment.

17. A: The only statement directly supported by the passage is choice A.

18. B: As used in this passage, the word "parasite" means an organism that lives on or in another organism, Choice B. Choice A and C are obviously wrong, since the passage mentions nothing of Paris or insects. Choice D is another definition for "parasite," but does not fit the context of the word used in this passage.

19. C: According to the description of Roundworms, they can live in the subcutaneous tissue of humans, Choice C. Choices A, B, and D describe where protozoa live and how they are transmitted.

20. D: According to the first paragraph, protozoa are transmitted through food and water contaminated by fecal matter. It can then be inferred that clean sanitary conditions will prevent the spread of protozoa, Choice D. Choice A is an incorrect inference because the passage discusses both larval and adult forms of parasites that infect humans. Choice B is an incorrect inference, since the first paragraph states that protozoa are transmitted by mosquitoes. Choice C is an incorrect inference because the second paragraph is about worms that infect humans.

21. D: To answer this question, you will need to verify all three statements in the passage. All three of these statements are true and are supported by the passage.

22. D: Since the passage describes superstitions from days gone by about treating asthma, answer choice D is the correct one. Answer choice A, asthma in the United States, is incorrect because even though that is mentioned in the first sentence, it is not the main idea. Answer choice B, methods of treating asthma, is not the best choice since it is vague about whether the methods are current or from long ago. Answer choice C, old wives tales, might have been a choice if old wives' tales had been mentioned in the passage, but it is not the best choice.

23. A: The reader can infer from the opening sentence that if so many people have asthma today, many would probably have had asthma long ago as well. Even though the environment today is different than it was long ago, people would still have suffered from the condition. The sentence explains why people long ago may have needed to try homemade methods of treating the condition.

24. B: The purpose of the passage is to describe different measures that people took for asthma long ago, before the advent of modern medicine. Answer choice A, herbal remedies, is incorrect because the majority of the "medicine" described in the passage is not herbal. The passage does not, as in answer choice C, define superstitions. Nor does it praise modern medicine, as answer choice D suggests.

25. A: Of all the choices listed, only answer choice A is an example of misusing a drug. It is listed as one of the ways that drugs are misused in the middle of the passage. Taking more or less of a prescription drug than the amount that the doctor ordered can be harmful to one's health. The other answer choices are not examples of misuse, nor do they appear in the passage. Make sure all of your answer choices are based on the passage given rather than information you may know or assume from other sources.

26. D: The passage does not say that ALL drugs add longevity. It says that drugs that are healthy and used properly add longevity. The word *all* makes the statement untrue.

27. C: The second paragraph of the passage notes that "up to one-third of people with peanut allergies have severe reactions." Since one-third is approximately 33%, (C) is the correct choice.

28. D: The second paragraph of the passage notes that in 2008, Duke experts stated that they expect to offer treatment in five years. Five years from 2008 is 2013.

29. B: The last sentence in paragraph five lists the cuisines in which one should watch for peanuts. Italian is not listed.

30. A: The second sentence of the first paragraph states that peanut allergy is the most common cause of food-related death.

31. C: The passage implies that it is not always easy to know which foods have traces of peanuts in them and that it's important to make sure you know what you're eating. This is hard or impossible if you share someone else's food.

32. D: Paragraph two gives examples of symptoms of peanut allergies and, more specifically, examples of symptoms of anaphylaxis. A running or stuffy nose is given as a symptom of the former, but not of the latter.

33. B: Hunter Gatherer is not a name the passage gives for a diet.

34. B: Dairy is listed as a food that is not allowed on the diet.

35. A: The passage notes that the idea behind the diet is that we are genetically adapted to the diet of our Paleolithic forebears.

36. B: The last sentence of the passage states that some studies support the idea of positive health benefits from the diet.

37. D: The directions indicate "for relief of headaches."

38. C: In this context upset means physical disorder.

39. C: The maximum one should take is 4 in a 24-hour period. One can call a doctor after 24 hours.

40. B: In this context, persists means continues.

41. B: Since one can take 1 pill every 4 hours, the answer is 3.

42. B: Tip number 2 best answers this detail question. The tip recommends that those who drink whole milk gradually switch to fat-free milk. Since the question asks about ways to reduce saturated fat and calories, using skim milk in the place of water does not address the issue being raised.

43. A: The author uses headings to organize the passage. While the headings are bold print, such font is not used to organize the passage (i.e. notify the reader of what information is forthcoming), but rather to draw the reader's eyes to the headings.

44. C: Tip number 2 bests answers this detail question. Reduced fat milk contains 2% fat.

45. B: Statement I and Statement II are both true statements about calcium rich foods. Canned fish, including salmon with bones, is recommended as a calcium rich food. Cheese is mentioned as a lactose-free alternative within the milk group. Statement III is false. According to the passage, condensed cream soups should be made with milk, not water.

46. D: The best choice for this question is choice (D). The other options would clarify information for minor details within the passage and would provide little new information for the reader. However, food recommendations for those who do not consume milk products are listed under a separate heading, and lactose intolerance is the only reason listed. The reader can deduce that this is a main idea in the passage and the definition of "lactose intolerance" would help explain this main idea to the reader.

47. D: The author's style is to give facts and details in a bulleted list. Of the options given, you are most likely to find this style in a health textbook. A tourist guidebook would most likely make recommendations about where to eat, not what to eat. An encyclopedia would list and define individual foods. A friendly letter would have a date, salutation, and a closing.

VocabularyandGeneralKnowledgeAnswer Key and Explanations

1. B: The best definition for the word *latent* is *dormant*. Something that is *latent* is unapparent but not necessarily nonexistent. For instance, a health condition can be latent without manifesting serious problems for many years. The word *thorough* suggests something that is complete and exhaustive, and this has no immediate connection to the word *latent*. The word *current* goes against the indication of the word *latent*, as the latter suggests something waiting for future events. The word *obvious* is an antonym of the word *latent*.

2. D: The meaning of the word *precipitous* is *abrupt*. A *precipitous* change in health is immediate and unexpected; in other words, it happens *abruptly*. The words *cautious*, *languid*, and *subtle* function largely as antonyms to the word *precipitous*, as all three words indicate something that occurs slowly or without obvious results.

3. C: The best definition for the word *recur* is *return*. A *recurring* problem is one that keeps coming back. While something that recurs happens again (and again), this does not suggest the same meaning as *redo*, which indicates a complete do-over. Similarly, the word *recreate* indicates not another occurrence but a totally new start. And while it is possible to see a connection between a condition that *recurs* and one that *revolves*, the question asks for the *best* definition. In this case, *return* is closest in meaning to *recur*, and *revolve* has too close a meaning to literal circular action to be the best definition in this case.

4. A: To *diffuse* is to *disseminate*, or spread around. The word *compress* suggests making something smaller and thus means the very opposite of *diffuse* and functions as an antonym. The word *distinct*, which means *unique* or *having qualities all its own*, has little similarity to the word *diffuse*. And while something might be *widened* to create a *diffusion*, the two words suggest related activities (or cause and effect) instead of similar meanings.

5. B: Something *anterior* is located near the *front*, so answer choice B offers the correct meaning of the word. Something *previous* comes before, but that does not necessarily mean the *front*. The word *crucial* has little relationship in meaning to the word *anterior*. The word *final* suggests the *end*, which is the very opposite of the *anterior*.

6. D: The word *insidious* suggests something that is sneaky, unobtrusive, and *subtle*. An *insidious* disease is difficult to identify, diagnose, and treat. The word *reliable* indicates *trustworthy*, which in some contexts would represent the very opposite of *insidious*. The word *limited* has no immediate connection to the word *insidious*, and the word *rapid* suggests speed and even ease of recognition— both of which are the opposite of *insidious*.

7. A: In this case, the best definition for the word *comply* is *follow*. To *comply* is to go along with a request, or to *follow* orders or expectations. The word *affect* suggests a causal relationship, but this is not the same as a synonym. (For instance, to *comply* might be to *affect* something positively.) It might be possible to *depend* on someone or something to *comply*, but once again the relationship between the words is causal, so the words cannot have the same meaning. To *decline* is to refuse to *follow* a request/demand, so this is the opposite of *comply*.

8. A: The context of the sentence suggests that the CEO intends to show that he is still in charge, in spite of leadership problems. As a result, the word *maintain* offers the best synonym for *assert*. The words *prevent* and *censure* would indicate that the CEO is blocking his own authority, and this goes against the tone of the sentence. The word *accept* is positive regarding the CEO's authority, but it makes no sense for him to accept his own authority; that is for the employees to do (or not to do) after he has *asserted* it.

9. C: To *occlude* is to block, hinder, or *prevent*. The word *release* suggests the very opposite of *occlude* (as something that is released cannot be simultaneously blocked). The word *invade* also indicates an opposite within certain contexts. (For instance, a virus cannot *invade* cells if measures have been taken to *occlude* it.) The word *direct*, which indicates an order or command as a verb, has no clear relationship with the word *occlude*.

10. A: The sentence suggests that the colleague's remarks went beyond silly or unnecessary. If Eirinn feels that she should file a formal complaint, the colleague's remarks must have been *inappropriate*. If the comments were either *delicate* or *friendly*, Eirinn would almost certainly not be upset by them. The colleague might very well have delivered the *untoward* comments in an *eager* way, but eagerness alone is not unacceptable. The suggestion of offense is what leads Eirinn to pursue a formal complaint.

11. A: The best definition for the word *superficial* is *surface*. Something or someone that is *superficial* is focused only on appearances, or on what is on the *surface*. A wound that is *superficial* concerns only the *surface* of the skin. The word *backward* has little connection to the word *superficial*, even as an antonym. A *superficial* person, or even a *superficial* injury, might create problems that are *awkward*, but this is not the meaning of the word itself. Something that is *superficial* tends to be fairly empty in meaning or behavior and thus could not be described as *intense*.

12. D: The best definition for the word *inverted* is *reversed*. To *invert* is to turn inside out or show a different side, and the same could be said for something that is *reversed*. The word *credible* suggests believability, and this has no clear connection to *inversion*. The word *benign* means lacking in danger, and there is no immediate relationship between the meaning of *inversion* and the potential for danger. The word *forward* is directional, and this could be seen as an antonym for *inverted*: to *invert* is to present a different side, whereas something that is *forward* is likely showing its correct side(s).

13. A: The meaning of the word *void* is *emit*. *Voiding* is the process of releasing or removing the contents of something. *Emitting* is also releasing or sending out something. This is the closest meaning among the answer choices. To *determine* is to make a decision or make up one's mind about something. This has almost nothing to do with *voiding*. To *confirm* is to approve or agree. Again, there is no connection to the word *void* in this. The word *prevent* might be seen as a type of antonym in that *voiding* is releasing, while *preventing* is retaining. At the same time, the word *prevent* requires a context that is not essential with the word *void*, so these two words as well have little connection.

14. C: The context of the sentence suggests that Catriona is concerned about the danger of the fever, so it can be inferred that the word *adverse* means *negative*. Most people try to prevent fevers before they occur, and taking the child to the doctor once the fever has set in cannot be described as *preventive*. The word *auspicious* suggests something positive, and this contradicts the meaning inherent to the sentence. The word *reckless*, while negative in context, is not as closely related to *adverse* as the actual word *negative*. In fact, *reckless* suggests a deliberate attempt to do something dangerous, while the sentence suggests that Catriona is trying to prevent something dangerous.

15. A: The meaning of the word *contingent* is *dependent*. *Contingency* indicates a relationship between two (or more) items or events. For instance, going on vacation might be *contingent* upon not catching the flu. As this suggests *dependency*, answer choice A is correct. The connotation of the word *contingent* has little to do with *protection*, so answer choice B cannot be correct. The word *definite* suggests something that is absolute and unquestioned, whereas the word *contingent* suggests only possibility. The items or events that have inherent *contingencies* might very well be *intended*, but the word *intended* does not have the necessary suggestion of *dependency* to be correct.

16. B: Philippa is upset that her plans to leave the hospital early are foiled, so she wants the doctor to explain himself. In other words, she wants his *justification* for the decision. The word *description* indicates what the doctor will be doing (that is, *describing* his reasons), but this does not indicate fully that Philippa is looking more for a clear explanation of the doctor's *reasoning* rather than a mere *description*. The doctor might be *persistent* in his refusal to let Philippa leave the hospital early, but this is *why* she wants a *rationale* and does little to define the word *rationale*. It is *ambiguity* that Philippa does *not* want; the context suggests that she expects a clear explanation from the doctor.

17. D: The best definition for the word *patent* is *unconcealed*. Something that is *patent* is open, obvious, clear, and leaving no doubt. The word *inconspicuous*, suggesting something subtle or less obvious, means the very opposite of *patent*. The word *privileged* has no clear relationship to the word *patent*. Something that is *patent* might also be *carelessly* so, but this suggests a context that is not implied in the actual meaning of the word.

18. C: The best definition for the word *labile* is *fluctuating*. *Lability* indicates an ability to change quickly and rapidly, and the word *fluctuating* suggests constant movement or change. The word *external* is related to appearance or behavior, and while both of these might be *labile*, the underlying context of the word *external* has little relationship with the word *labile*. The word *meticulous* suggests the very opposite of the word *labile*. Something or someone *meticulous* is patient and takes the time to do something carefully and/or correctly. *Lability* indicates impatience more than *meticulousness*. The word *integral* indicates an inherent quality, and while *lability* might very well be *integral* to some things, the word *labile* means change, and the word *integral* does not.

19. B: The best definition for the word *impending* is *approaching*. An *impending* event is soon to arrive, and the word *approaching* indicates that something is on its way. The *impending* event might also be *demanding* on one's time or energy, but something *demanding* is not necessarily *impending*, so the relationship between the two words is too conditional. Something *impending* might also be *perilous*, and in literary terms it is often that *impending* events connote negative results. But the question asks for the *best* definition, and this is *approaching*. The word *producing* has little connection to the word *impending*, so answer choice D is incorrect.

20. A: The meaning of the word *exacerbate* is *aggravate*. To *exacerbate* is to make something worse, and this is the very connotation of the word *aggravate*. To *exaggerate* is to suggest an extreme that does not exist, and as the word *exacerbate* indicates the potential for this very extreme answer choice B cannot be correct. The word *outrage* is specifically related to anger, and while something that *exacerbates* might also *outrage,* there is too much of a condition for a human response in answer choice C. For instance, an injury, illness, or health condition can be *exacerbated*, but it cannot be *outraged*. To *alleviate* is to make something better, the very opposite of *exacerbate*.

21. B: The meaning of the word *lethargic* is *sluggish*. Something or someone *lethargic* is lacking in energy. *Lethargy* might produce a sense of *calm*, but it is often a false calm that results from the lack of energy rather than an inherent quality of the condition. Something or someone *lethargic* might very well be *conscious*, but this can be said of those who are not *lethargic* as well. The word *elaborate* suggests a sophistication that has no direct connection to the meaning of the word *lethargic*.

22. D: The context of the sentence suggests that the lie is anything but a good one, so the truth is clear, and the meaning of the word *overt* is *obvious*. The lie might be *unnecessary*, but this does not capture the same meaning as *obvious*. The word *tangible* suggests something that can be touched, and this cannot be said of a lie—although Niamh sees the *tangible* results of her son's lie. Niamh's son might be *energetic* in telling this lie, but the word *energetic* is not closely related enough in meaning to the word *overt*.

23. D: The best definition for the word *discrete* is *separate*. Something that is *discrete* is distinct, detached, or on its own. The word *standard* suggests a customary quality, and this has no immediate connection to the word *discrete*. Similarly, the word *normal* indicates something that is typical or usual, and there is no relationship between this and the word *discrete*. The word *subtle* indicates caution, something that is done in an inconspicuous way. Something that is *discrete* might also be *subtle* (as well as *standard* or *normal*), but these are outside qualities that have no effect on the inherent meaning of the word *discrete*.

24. C: The best definition for the word *adsorb* is *accumulate*. To *adsorb* is to gather (such as particles) on the surface of something. Whereas *absorb* suggests a permeation, *adsorb* suggests an accumulation. The word *divide* indicates the very opposite of the word *adsorb*, since the process of *adsorption* gathers together. The word *process* has no immediate connection to the word *adsorb*. While *adsorption* is itself a *process, adsorbing* does not usually result in *processing* the particles that are gathered. Also, what is *adsorbed* might also be *contained*, but the suggestion of *containment* is conditional on other elements and not necessarily a part of the underlying meaning of the word *adsorb*.

25. B: The best definition for the word *compensatory* is *offsetting*. To *compensate* is to make up for something—in other words, to *offset* whatever is missing. Something *compensatory* might also be *corrupted*, but the presence of corruption has little to do with the meaning of the word *compensatory*. The word *varying* suggests change or fluidity, and this has no immediate connection to the word *compensatory*. The word *contradictory* indicates going against what is expected, and again this has no clear relationship with the meaning of *compensatory*.

26. A: The word *incompatible* suggests that two or more things cannot go together—that they are *conflicting*. The word *subsequent* suggests an event in which one thing follows another. The word *relevant* indicates that two things are related or appropriate for one another, so this could function as an antonym to *incompatible*. Similarly, the word *suitable* suggests that two things go together, so this is an antonym.

27. C: The word *lateral* indicates something that is sideways or *sideward*. There is no clear relationship between this and the word *positive*. The word *central* indicates a location other than the side, so it cannot be correct. The word *serious* suggests a quality about the word *lateral*, that a *lateral* injury can be *serious*, but this requires a qualification of the original word.

28. D: Something that is *distended* is *bulging* beyond its expected boundaries. The word *embellished* indicates that something has been adorned, and there is no immediate relationship between this and *distended*. The word *abridged* functions as a kind of antonym, because something that is *abridged* has been *reduced*. In the same way, something that is *tightened* is pulled in, the very opposite of being *distended*.

29. C: The word *exiguous* suggests a lack or *inadequacy*. The word *superfluous* indicates an excessive amount, so this is an antonym for *exiguous*. The word *defective* indicates a failure, but this is not the same thing as a lack. A *defective* action can create an *exiguous* result, but this is a cause-and-effect relationship instead of a similarity in meaning. The word *eager* has no clear relationship with the word *exiguous*.

30. B: A claim that is *untenable* is *groundless* or without any support. The very opposite of an *untenable* claim would be a *logical* one, so answer choice A is an antonym. Something that is *opaque* is lacking in any transparency: there is no immediate relationship between *opaque* and *untenable*, except that an *untenable* claim could potentially be *opaque* as well. These are, however, entirely different qualities. Something *analogous* is similar or compatible, but there is nothing immediate in this to connect it with the word *untenable*.

31. D: To *placate* is to *comfort* or bring peace to someone or something. To *authorize* is to approve, so these words have no connection to each other in meaning. To *incite* is to create anger, so this is the very opposite of *placate*. To *clarify* is to make clear in explanation or meaning. As with *authorize*, there is nothing direct in the meaning to connect these words with each other.

32. A: To *inure* is to *toughen* someone or something against a current or future event. To *pretend* is to create an element of fantasy. While this is not a direct antonym to *inure*, there is a potential connection in opposites: something that is *inured* cannot *pretend* to ignore circumstances and must accept reality. To *anticipate* is to expect something to occur. One can *anticipate* an event by being *inured* to it, but this is a series of actions rather than a suggestion of a synonymous relationship. To *forget* is to lose track of something; a person who is *inured* cannot be allowed to *forget*.

33. C: The word *clement* indicates a situation (or individual) that is beneficent or *favorable*. In terms of opposites, *inclement* weather is bad weather that does not bode well for outdoor activities. Being *clement* means *not* being *difficult* or *angry*, so both answer choices are incorrect. A person who is *clement* can also be *righteous* in behavior, but the latter suggests a result of the former, indicating a cause-and-effect relationship instead of a relationship of synonyms.

34. A: To *malign* is to *harm* in a serious way. To *submit* is to give in and obey an order or expectation. There is no clear relationship between this and *malign*, so the words cannot be synonyms. To *improve* is to make better; to *malign* is to make worse, so the words are antonyms. To *conceive* is to create, so there is no direct relationship between this and *malign*.

35. B: To exist in *synergy* is to exist in a state of dwelling together comfortably or living in *harmony*. To *delay* is to prevent or slow down, and there is no immediate connection between this and *synergy*. A situation of *distress* indicates conflict, so this cannot be a state of *synergy*. A *hindrance* indicates a block, and this is the opposite of *synergy*.

36. D: To *recede* is to pull back or *retreat*. It can also suggest a diminishment, which would make the word *increase* an antonym. To *dilate* also indicates an increase or expansion, so this functions almost as an opposite. To *present* is to give or offer, and this has no clear connection with *recede*.

37. A: To *inflame* is to aggravate suddenly. For instance, banging an already sore knee could *inflame* the discomfort. As a result, the best definition is the word *worsen*. The word *ignite* has the hint of fire that is suggested by *inflame*, but in the latter case the word suggests a metaphorical condition or situation rather than anything connected literally to a flame. What is more, the word *ignite*, when metaphorical, indicates a cause (i.e., to *ignite* someone's interest), but it has no immediate connection to making something worse. To *lull* is the soothe or make better, so this is an antonym for *inflame*. To *inflame* something could be to *endanger* someone, but the relationship is causal rather than synonymous.

38. A: A *detriment* is a *drawback*, something negative that keeps a condition or situation from being as good as it should or could be. For instance, a cold could be a *detriment* for someone who hopes to enjoy a vacation. The word *retribution* suggests payback for some wrong that has been done, but there is no direct connection in this to a *drawback*—except that the *retribution* will almost certainly be a *drawback* for whoever is on the receiving end. The word *excitement* suggests eagerness or enthusiasm, and it is unlikely that a *detriment* could foster such an emotion. An *indulgence* is an excess of some kind (either of something tangible or of approval for behavior), and this suggests the very opposite of *detriment*—unless the *indulgence* ultimately represents a *detriment*, but that is causal and not indicated in the actual meaning.

39. C: The word *turgid* means swollen or *inflated*. This is not to be confused with *turbid*, which means *murky* (answer choice B). The word *intricate* suggests complexity, and there is nothing within the word *turgid* to indicate an immediate connection to this. The word *acceptable* means that something is good, and the word *turgid* reflects a condition that is unnatural or potentially serious, so answer choice D cannot be correct.

40. C: The word *paucity* indicates a *lack* or scarcity of something. The word *hunger* indicates a close possible meaning, in that hunger is the result of a *paucity* of food. But the word *result* in that statement indicates the real relationship, which requires a further explanation not immediate in the meaning. (In other words, *hunger* might result from *paucity*, but *paucity* does not always mean that the *lack* is one of food.) The word *affluence* suggests wealth or excess, so this functions as an antonym. The word *insistence* suggests an ongoing determination that something should be or occur, so there is no immediate connection in meaning to *paucity*.

41. D: To *proscribe* is to *forbid* something. This is the very opposite of *prescribe*, which is to recommend or encourage. A doctor might *proscribe* excess salt and *prescribe* blood pressure medication. To *belittle* is to insult someone or tear him/her down with negative comments. This has almost nothing to do with the meaning of *proscribe*, so this answer choice cannot be correct. To *increase* is to add, and since the meaning of *proscribe* suggests some form of reduction, there is a hint of an antonym in this word (although the relationship is ultimately causal—to *proscribe* might lead to a decrease). To *praise* is to show approval, and this again is the opposite meaning embedded in *proscribe*.

42. B: The word *austere* suggests meagerness or something/someone *stark* in choices, attitude, or behavior. The word *calm* is related to a condition of quietness, and while someone or something *austere* might also be *calm*, there is not enough in the meaning of each word to suggest a clear relationship. The word *dependable* indicates someone or something that can be relied upon. Again, there is not enough in the meaning to indicate a synonym with *austere*. The word *greedy* suggests a desire for excess, and this is the very opposite of the suggestion in *austere*.

43. D: To *delineate* is to *detail* something clearly. A mother who *delineates* instructions presents them so that her child knows exactly what to do. The very opposite of *delineate* would be *confuse*, since the goal of *delineating* is to avoid *confusion*. There is no clear connection in meaning with either *open* (as a verb) or *brag*.

44. B: Something *expedient* offers the best or most *practical* solution. The word *grateful* indicates a thankfulness for something, and there is nothing in this meaning to connect it with the meaning of *expedient*. Something *unprofitable* has no value, and this is the opposite of *expedient*, as the word *expedient* suggests a solution that is intended to offer immediate value. The word *substitute*, in suggesting an alternative, has a causal relationship with *expedient*: the *expedient* decision might also be the *substitute* option, but there is not enough in the meaning to make this direct connection.

45. B: To *facilitate* is to make something easier, or to *smooth* the way for something to occur. To *recast* is to start over; to *decide* is to make a choice. Neither of these has a direct relationship with the meaning of *facilitate*, so both are incorrect. To *thwart* is to hinder or make something difficult. This is opposite in meaning to *facilitate*.

46. C: The word *restive* describes someone who is *tense* about something and thus moving around (rather than resting comfortably). Someone who is *restive* might also be *frightened*, but he or she can also just be fidgety, so there is not enough suggestion of *fear* in *restive* to justify answer choice A. Someone who is *restive* might be so as the result of *hostility*, but this is a causal relationship instead of a synonymous one. Someone who is *apathetic* does not care about what is happening, and this indicates an opposite meaning of the word *restive*.

47. C: To have a *recourse* is to have another *option*. In other words, a *recourse* suggests a way out of a situation or an alternative choice. To *ambush* is to attack in surprise, so there is no real connection here to the meaning of *recourse*. An *obligation* is a required action, and a *recourse* is an alternative one, so these words suggest opposite meanings. A *proposal* is a presented idea, and while the *recourse* might come as the result of a *proposal* from someone, this is a cause-and-effect relationship.

48. A: To know the *impetus* for one's actions is to understand his or her *motivation(s)*, or reasons for doing something. A *diversion* is a distraction, so there is no clear relationship between this and the meaning of *impetus*. The word *authority* suggests a right of power, and again there is nothing in this to indicate the meaning of *impetus*. A *prevention* keeps one from doing something or keep something from occurring. There is nothing in this meaning to connect it to the meaning of *impetus*.

49. D: To know the *salient* points is to know what is *important*. The meaning of *salient* suggests information that is essential, and this goes beyond the meaning of *acceptable* (as allowable or adequate). Something *ordinary* is commonplace and does not indicate the degree of *importance* suggested in the meaning of *salient*. The word *peripheral* suggests the quality of being marginal or unimportant, so this is the opposite of *salient*.

50. C: Someone who is *laconic* tends to be *brief* in speech, getting right to the point and saying little else. Being *laconic*, or brief, is not the same as being *slow*, however, so the words do not have a close relationship in meaning. Being *laconic* also does not mean being *incomplete*: someone can be brief without leaving out important information. The word *tidy*, with its suggestion of cleanliness and organization, has no real connection to the meaning of *laconic*.

Grammar Answer Key and Explanations

1. A: Volleyball is a team sport that follows the verb "to play," whereas individual sports like yoga follow the verb "to do."

2. D: The word "every" is a singular noun and should be followed by a singular pronoun. In this case, the only singular pronoun is "her."

3. A: The phrasal verb "to put up with" means to have to deal with something or someone.

4. D: The future tense is will + the infinitive, in this case "will study."

5. B: This should be an adverb, and the correct spelling is "sympathetically."

6. A: The subject of this sentence, "a team," is singular, so the verb also should be singular.

7. B: This sentence is in the past tense so the phrasal verb should also be in the past tense.

8. B: The correct spelling is "presents."

9. D: The correct spelling is "authority."

10. B: The possessive for "each" is singular. The only singular possessive choice is B: her.

11. A: The word needed here is an adverb. Tearfully is the best choice.

12. B: Choice B: gives the correct spelling.

13. C: The correct choice must complete the future perfect form. Bring is the correct choice.

14. C: Each requires a singular possessive. The only singular possessive form is "his".

15. B: The verb tense of this sentence needs to be in the past.

16. B: The correct choice must be an adverb; well is the correct choice.

17. C: The correct spelling is niece.

18. D: The correct spelling is judgment.

19. B: The pronoun *Everyone* is singular and thus needs a singular verb. Among the verbs provided, only *needs* is both singular and makes sense in the context of the sentence. Stripped of the dependent clause, the sentence reads, "Everyone needs to see the new Manet exhibit." The verbs *should* and *must* both become unreadable with the addition of the infinitive phrase "to see" (while both would work if the "to" were removed), and the verb *have* is plural.

20. A: The possessive pronoun *Their* at the beginning of the sentence suggests third-person plurality, so answer choices B and D are immediately incorrect. (The first-person use of *we* and *I* excludes them as options.) The real choice comes down to *he and she* or *him and her*. In the sentence, the blank falls just after the start of a dependent clause, and this blank represents the subject of the dependent clause. As a result, the subjective case *he and she* must be correct.

21. B: After hearing about the party, Desmond knows that he *should have gone*. The expression *should have went* is never correct, under any circumstances. The expression *should go* makes little sense, as the context of the sentence indicates that the party has already occurred. The expression *should have been* also makes little sense, as the sentence indicates that Desmond wanted to *attend* the party, not *be* the party.

3 HESI Admission Assessment Practice Tests

22. C: The word *who* is always used when referring to individual people, and the context of the sentence suggests that Loman is phoning a singular person *who* is the organizer. The word *that* is appropriate for groups, and the word *which* is appropriate for inanimate objects or things. The word *this* makes virtually no sense when added to the blank in the sentence.

23. D: Clearly, the cat belongs to the Millers, so it can be said to be *theirs* in the sentence. The context indicates that the cat is not Nessa's, so it is not *hers*. The Millers are clearly plural, so the cat is not *his*, singular. And as there is no first-person indication in the sentence, the cat cannot be *ours*. No doubt, that is what the Millers would say, but because the sentence is third-person (and has no dialogue) the shift to first person is not appropriate here.

24. B: The presence of the conjunction *or* indicates the need for a singular verb. This sentence can be broken down with only one of the names to read correctly: "See to it that Derek <u>collects</u>..." or "See to it that Una <u>collects</u>..." The verb *are collecting* makes no sense when placed in the sentence. The plural verb *collect* does not work with the singular context implied by *or*. The verb *would collect* almost works but ultimately sounds strange when placed in the sentence.

25. A: The blank requires a second subject for the sentence, and the pronoun *she* is in the subjective case. The pronouns *him* and *me* are both in the objective case and thus do not fit the sentence correctly. It should be noted that the pronoun *they* is also subjective, but it is plural and thus does not fit the singular verb *knows*. While *Neither...nor...* is considered a singular expression, it can take a plural verb when the second subject is plural.

26. D: Because *was* is a <u>being verb</u> (those including *am, is, are, was, were*, etc.), it requires a subjective case pronoun to follow it. So, instead of "It was *him*," the expression is correctly "It was *he*." The possessive pronoun *his* makes no sense in the context of the sentence, and the reflexive *himself* could only follow the original pronoun. (For instance, "It was *he himself*." As this sounds fairly awkward, *himself* has no real place in this sentence.)

27. C: In this context, the word in the blank is the subject of the dependent clause and thus should be in the subjective case. Only *whoever* fits this requirement. To know for sure, simply substitute *whoever* with *he/she* and *whomever* with *him/her*. "He arrives first / she arrives first" makes far more sense than "him arrives first / her arrives first." So what about just using *who*? While technically in the subjective case, *who* sounds strange in the sentence, while *whoever* makes more sense. Why say, "The grand prize of $10,000 will be given to *who* arrives at the finish line first," when you can say, "The grand prize of $10,000 will be given to *whoever* arrives at the finish line first."

28. A: The blank in the sentence requires only a single preposition to create a prepositional phrase: "*off* the roof." Doubling up on prepositions (*off of, off from, away from*) is incorrect.

29. B: The word *committee* is a collective noun that can take either a singular or plural verb, depending on the context of the sentence. If there is agreement in the committee, the word is singular; if there is disagreement in the committee, the word is plural. For example, "The committee *agrees*..." but "The committee *disagree*..." In this question, the committee *were* in disagreement.

30. B: This question asks for the correct past tense usage of the verb *drink* when affixed to the helping verb *had*. The verb *drink* conjugates accordingly: *drink, drank, had drunk*. With the use of *had*, the correct choice is *drunk*. Fortunately, *had drunken* is never correct.

31. D: This question asks for the correct past tense usage of the verb *see* with the helping verb *has*. The verb *see* conjugates as such: *see, saw, had seen*. In this sentence, the use of *has* can take the place of *had* to indicate the correct usage: "What no eye has *seen*..."

32. C: The context of the sentence indicates that the ice-cream man has not yet arrived. The sentence projects into the future to say that *when* he arrives the children *will be excited*. In the latter case, the verb also suggests a future context and is thus correct. The past tense *were excited* makes no sense in the sentence. The conditional tenses *would be excited* and *would have been excited* also make little sense in the context of future activities that are presented as definite.

33. A: This sentence requires a slightly unexpected combination of future and continuous past tenses. The speaker points out that when something happens in the future (i.e., the completion of the final pose), something will then have been in the process of occurring for two hours. In this case, the verb *will have been doing* successfully indicates both cases to make the sentence read correctly. The fully future *will do* and *will be doing* do not work without some hint of a continuous past sentence as well. The verb *would be doing* is conditional, but the rest of the context of the sentence does not have enough suggestion of conditional activity to make this verb work. The speaker is confident of completing the yoga routine; the verb needs to indicate this. (The use of *If* at the beginning of the sentence instead of *Once* would provide the sense of the conditional.)

34. A: The blank space requires the start of a dependent clause. In this case, the word *that* is most correct. The word *which* is more correct to introduce a clause that is not necessarily essential to the sentence. Because the sentence makes little sense without the clause, the word *that* is necessary to introduce it. The word *than* suggests comparison, so it has no place introducing a dependent clause. The word *who* should introduce a phrase or clause that refers to a person, and since the sentence refers to the inanimate *vacation plan*, the word *who* is not correct.

35. D: The sentence requires two adverbs: *really badly*. The adverb *badly* modifies the verb *performed*, while the adverb *really* modifies the adverb *badly* to answer the question *How?* All other answer choices are either entirely correct or only partially correct. The words *real* and *bad* are adjectives without the addition of *-ly*, so both cannot be correct to modify a verb and an adverb.

36. D: No preposition is necessary at the end of the question. The directional word *Where* indicates location, so the addition of *to*, *from*, or *at* is unnecessary and makes the sentence grammatically incorrect. What is more, the use of *from* and *at* makes little sense in the context of the question.

37. C: The verb *have* is correct here to complete the verb: *should have*. The entire expression is a verb, so the preposition *of* cannot be correct to complete it. The verb *be* makes no sense in the context of the sentence. The verb *has* does not fit the use of *I* or the addition of *should*. (The verb *should* always requires the form *have*; the form *has* is never correct with it.)

38. A: The comma belongs after the dependent clause, so it is correct between the words *mother* and *he*: *When Finn called his mother, he did not tell her about all of his plans.* The comma between *called* and *his* makes little sense, as there is no need for a pause between these words. In the same way, the comma between *not* and *tell* breaks the sentence up awkwardly, so it cannot be correct. The comma after the word *When* is incorrect because the comma belongs after the entire dependent clause instead of just after the relative adverb.

39. D: The context of the sentence indicates that Professor Howard is grading the papers of all thirty-five students, so the sentence requires the possessive of a plural word. The correct form would be *students'*. The form *student's* would suggest the possessive of a singular word. The word *students* is simply plural but not possessive, and the sentence indicates the possession of *papers* belonging to *students*. The form *student's* is never correct.

40. D: The sentence requires an adverb form to modify the verb *did*, and the only correct adverb form among the answer choices is *well*. The words *good* and *great* are adjectives. The word *worse* makes little sense as it contradicts the context of the sentence: most teachers do not praise their students for doing *worse* on something.

41. C: The comma belongs before the coordinating conjunction to indicate the combination of two independent clauses. In this case, the coordinating conjunction is *but*, so the correct version is: *Olaf planned to see the movie, but he could not go after he caught the flu.* The comma after the coordinating conjunction is never correct if there is no comma before the coordinating conjunction. (A comma after the coordinating conjunction is correct—when there is also one before it—if there is a required pause at the start of the new independent clause.) The comma between *movie* and *he* removes the conjunction *but* and thus functions as a comma splice, incorrectly joining two independent clauses. The semicolon between *but* and *he* makes no sense in its placement.

42. A: The single apostrophe is appropriate because the context of the sentence suggests that Melissa and Caroline share the dorm room. If they were in separate rooms, then the form *Melissa's and Caroline's* would be acceptable, but the sentence indicates that Maura only knocks on the door of one room. The form *Melissa's and Caroline* reads awkwardly by assigning the possession to the first person and leaving the reader unsure of what this means. The lack of apostrophes altogether also makes little sense by placing the two names in the middle of the sentence but not indicating clearly their relationship to the dorm room.

43. C: The form *1980s* is correct without the apostrophe, since it is plural instead of possessive. Any form with the apostrophe at the end (*1980's* and *1980s'*) is incorrect to indicate a plural form. The form with the apostrophe at the beginning of the expression (*'1980s*) would only be correct if the *19* were dropped at the beginning (*'80s*), because the apostrophe here suggests that something has been removed from the expression—much like a contraction.

44. C: The context of the sentence indicates contrast: Jean intended to hold the picnic, *but* the rain prevented it from happening. The conjunction *and* suggests addition that makes the sentence sound more confusing. The word *however* is not a conjunction and creates a run-on sentence when added just after a comma (and without a coordinating conjunction). The word *or* suggests the presence of options or alternatives, and this makes little sense in the context of the sentence.

45. B: If the instructor intends to prevent cheating, the study notes will have to be collected *before* the exam. Collecting them *during* or *after* the exam would only increase the potential for the students to consult them. (And the context of the sentence suggests that consulting the study notes would qualify as cheating.) Collecting the study notes *upon* the exam makes almost no sense. It would be possible to collect them *upon the start* of the exam, but as the sentence does not include the expression *the start*, the preposition *upon* does not work here.

46 C: This is a rare case when both forms of *effect* (verb and noun) are used correctly in the sentence. The word *effect* is used as a verb when it expresses a specific desire to cause something to occur: *effect* a compromise, *effect* a change. The noun form of *effect* is the result of the change, so both forms are correct in this sentence. The form *affect* is incorrect in both places in the sentence.

47. A: The context of the sentence suggests that Eleanora cannot *accept* (or receive) gifts, *except* (or only) from colleagues and only when the gift is a birthday gift. This requires that *accept* go in the first blank and *except* go in the second blank.

48. D: The form *ensure* indicates a desire to guarantee that something occurs. The form *insure* is related only to insurance. In other words, a homeowner will *insure* a home against fire to *ensure* that he or she is covered if a fire breaks out. Answer choice D places the forms in the correct order for the sentence: *ensure, insure.*

49. B: Since the second part of this sentence goes on to list examples that help support the point made in the first sentence, "for instance" is the best transitional phrase.

50. C: The second part of the sentence adds additional evidence to prove the claim made in the first part. "In fact" is the best transition to introduce supporting evidence.

MathematicsAnswer Key and Explanations

1. A: $(400 \times .25) = 100$

2. C: The reciprocal of a fraction is the inverse of the fraction. The fraction is turned up side down. $6 = {}^6/_1$, the reciprocal is ${}^1/_6$.

3. B: $145°F - 32°F = 113°F$, $113°F \div 4hrs = 28.25°F/hr$

4. A: $240 \div 6 = 40$, $6 \div 2 = 3$, (40 pcks of pens x $2.35 ea.) + (3 pcks of staplers x $12.95 ea.) = $132.85

5. D: $.45 \times 100 = 45\%$

6. B: 500mg Ca – 325 mg Ca = 175 mg Ca

7. C: Set up ratio of $4/5 = 20/x$, $4x = 20(5)$, $x = 100/4$, $x = 25$ mL dose

8. A: Moving right of the decimal point one space is the tenths position

9. C: $1.25 \times 100 = 125\%$

10. B: $12.8 \div 64 = .20$. $.20 = 20/100$, reduce $20/100$ to $1/5$

11. D: $300 \times .33 = 99$

12. D: $4/5 - 1/3$, find common denominator, $12/15 - 5/15 = 7/15$ cups

13. A: $3/4 - 1/2 = 3/4 - 2/4 = 1/4$

14. B: 48 students – 32 girls = 16 boys, $16 \div 48 = .33$, $.33 \times 100 = 33\%$

15. B: infant dose = (24 months ÷ 150) 15 mg = 2.4mg

16. C: $(15/2) - (43/8) = (60/8) - (43/8) = 17/8 = 2\ 1/8$

17. A: 20% is 1/5 of a number $1/5 = 35/x$. $1x = 35(5)$, $x = 175$

18. D: any number multiplied by 0 is equal to 0

19. B: 7.95 ÷1.5= 5.3, remember to move decimal point one place over before beginning equation

20. C: 7 Divided by 10 = .7

21. C: 4/8 reduced to ½, 1 divided by 2 = .5

22. A: –25, Add the positive and negative number together.

23. B: 41 Divided by 100 equals .41

24. B: This is a simple addition problem. Start with the ones column (on the right). Add the figures 8+1, 4+1, 2+3 to get the answer 559.

25. C: This is a simple addition problem with carrying. Start with the ones column and add 0+1. Write down the 1 and add the digits in the tens column: 8+3. Write down the 1 and add the 1 to the digits in the hundreds column. Add 9+1+1 and write down 1. Add the 1 to the digits in the thousands column. Add 3+7+1 and write down the 1. Add the 1 to the digits in the ten-thousands column. Add 1+1 and write down 2 to get the answer 21,011.

26. B: This is a simple subtraction problem. Start with the ones column and subtract 7-6, then 3-1, then 5-3, then 8-6 to get 2,221.

27. C: This is a multiplication problem with carrying. Start with the ones column. Multiply 2 by each digit above it beginning with the ones column. Write down each product: going across-- it will read 1268. Now multiply 7 by each of the digits above it. Write down each product: going across, the figure will read 4501. Ensure that the 1 is in the tens column and the other numbers fall evenly to the right. Now add the numbers like a regular addition problem to get 46,296.

28. D: This is a simple division problem. Divide 63 into 181. It goes in 2 times. Write 2 above the 1 and subtract 136 from 181. The result is 55. Bring down the 4. Divide 63 in 554. It goes in 8 times. Write 8 above the first 4 and subtract 504 from 554 to get 50. Bring down the 4. Divide 63 into 504. It goes in 8 times.

29. C: This is a simple addition problem. Line up the decimals so that they are all in the same place in the equation, and see that there is a 3 by itself in the hundredths column. Then add the tenths column: 6+3+5 to get 14. Write down the 4 and carry the 1. Add the ones column: 3 plus the carried 1. Write down 4. Then write down the 1.

30. D: This is multiplication with decimals. Multiply 3 by 9 to get 27. Put down the 7 and carry the 2. Multiply 3 by 1 to get 3. Add the 2. Write 5 to the left of 5. Multiply the 2 by the 9 to get 18. Enter the 8 and carry 1. Multiply 2 by 1 to get 2. Add 1 and write down 3. Add the two lines together, making sure that the 8 in the bottom figure is even with the 5. Get 437. Count 4 decimal points over (2 from the top multiplier and 2 from the second multiplier) and add a 0 before adding the decimal.

31. C: To solve, divide .08 into .3. Move the decimal in .08 over 2 places to make it an 8. Because this decimal point was moved 2 places, it must be done to the other decimal too. .3 becomes 30.0. Now divide 8 into 30. Put a 3 above 0 (ensure that the decimal is beside it) and subtract 24 from 30. Bring down the 0 and put it beside the 6. Divide 8 into 60. Put 7 above the 0 and subtract 56 from 60. Bring down the 0 and put it beside the 4. Divide 8 into 40. Put 5 beside the 7.

32. C: Count from the 5: tenths, hundredths, thousandths.

33. A: This is a simple subtraction problem involving decimals. Line up the decimals and subtract 7 from 3. Since 7 is a larger number than 3, borrow ten from the 4. Cross out the 4 and make it 3. Now subtract 7 from 13 to get 6. Subtract 1 from 3 and get 2. Place the decimal point before the 2.

34. D: Circle the 4 in the hundredths place. Look at the digit in the thousandths place. Since that digit is more than 5, the 4 is rounded up becoming a 5.

35. A: To add fractions, ensure that the denominator (the number on the bottom) is always the same common denominator. Since there is not common denominator in this case, change both fractions to 14ths. 1/2 equals 7/14. 1/7 equals 2/14. Now add the whole numbers: 2+3 = 5 and the resulting fraction become 9/14.

36. B: To subtract fractions, ensure that the denominator (the number on the bottom) is the same. Having the same "common denominator" is essential to solving the problem. Since there is no common denominator in this case, t, change both fractions to 36ths. 1/9 equals 4/36. 1/4 equals 9/36. The equation now looks like this: $3\frac{4}{36} - 1\frac{9}{36}$. Change the 3 to 2 and add 36 to the numerator (the top number) so that the fractions can be subtracted. The equation now looks like this: $2\frac{40}{36} - 1\frac{9}{36}2$. Subtract: $1\frac{31}{36}$

37. A: To multiply mixed numbers, you must first create improper fractions. Multiply the whole number by the denominator, and then add the numerator.

$$3\frac{1}{8} \text{ becomes } \frac{25}{8}$$

The problem will look like this: $\frac{28}{5} x \frac{19}{3} x \frac{12}{5} = \frac{5700}{120} = 47\frac{1}{2}$

38. A: To divide fractions, change the second fraction to its reciprocal (its reverse) and multiply: $\frac{1}{8} x \frac{5}{4}$

39. B: The denominator has been multiplied by 4 to get 20. Think of what number multiplied by 4 totals 12.

40. C: Divide the numerator and denominator by 17.

41. A: Since all the answers have a 7 as the whole number, multiply 7 x 14. The answer is 98. The remainder is 1.

42. D: Divide 3 by 50 to get .06 or 6%.

43. C: Divide 60 by 5 to get 12. Multiply 12 by 3.

44. A: Rewrite the problem as 40 x .5% and solve. Since the answer choices are not in percent form, do not forget to divide by 100 to convert from percentage to decimal.

45. D: Divide 2 by 10 (not 10 by 2). Multiply by 100 to get answer in % form.

46. C: To change a fraction to a percent, multiply it by 100:
$$\frac{3}{5} x \frac{100}{1}$$

47. A: To solve, first write the fraction as $\frac{15}{100}$. Reduce by dividing numerator and denominator both by 5.

48. B: To solve change 1 ¼% to a decimal: .0125. Now add an x for the question mark:
$.0125x = 1.5$. Divide 1.5 by .0125.

49. C: To solve, rewrite the equation with a decimal in place of the percent:
8=0.25x

$$x = \frac{8}{.25} = \frac{800}{25} = 32$$

50. C: To solve, change the percent to a decimal:
$$.40x = 18$$
$$x = \frac{18}{.40} = \frac{1800}{40} = 45$$

BiologyAnswer Key and Explanations

1. A: All organisms begin life as a single cell.

2. B: The process by which organisms use energy is called metabolism.

3. D: Only cells with a membrane around the nucleus are called eukaryotes.

4. C: The two types of cellular transport are active (which requires the cell to invest energy) and passive (which does not require the cell to expend energy).

5. A: Aerobic means in the presence of oxygen.

6. B: When both parents give offspring the same allele, the offspring is homozygous for that particular trait.

7. C: Genetics is the study of heredity.

8. B: Scientists suggest that evolution has occurred through a process called natural selection.

9. D: The cellular hierarchy starts with the cell, the simplest structure, and progresses to organisms, the most complex structures.

10. B: A hypertonic solution is a solution with a higher particle concentration than in the cell, and consequently lower water content than in the cell. Water moves from the cell to the solution, causing the cell to experience water loss and shrink.

11. C: Interphase is the period when the DNA is replicated (or when the chromosomes are replicated) and is the longest part of the cell cycle.

12. B: Recessive alleles are represented by lower case letters, while dominant alleles are represented by upper case letters,

13. C: Dominant genes are always expressed when both alleles are dominant (BB) or when one is dominant and one is recessive (Bg). In this case, ¾ or 75% will have brown eyes.

14. A: The trait Ll describes the genotype of the person or the traits for the genes they carry. It is heterozygous because it contains a dominant gene and a recessive gene. Tallness is the phenotype of the person or the physical expression of the genes they carry, because L for tallness is the dominant gene.

15. C: Arthritis is a type of non-communicable disease because it is not passed from person to person.

16. D: All living organisms on Earth utilize the same triplet genetic code, in which a three-nucleotide sequence called a codon provides information corresponding to a particular amino acid to be added to a protein. In contrast, many organisms, especially certain types of bacteria, do not use oxygen. These organisms live in oxygen-poor environments, and may produce energy through fermentation. Other organisms may live in dark environments, such as in caves or deep underground. Many organisms reproduce asexually by budding or self-fertilization, and only the most evolutionarily-advanced organisms make use of neurotransmitters in their nervous systems.

17. B: The nitrogenous bases found in DNA are thymine, guanine, adenine, and cytosine. Uracil is the base used in mRNA in the place of thymine.

18. A: Water is a polar substance and so does not interact well with nonpolar compounds (think: oils). Enzymes are actually an example of tertiary proteins not secondary. Exergonic reactions create energy, rather than use it up.

19. C: Ribosomes are small intracellular organelles that build proteins. The proteins are then sent to the Golgi apparatus for modification and packaging into their final form. The endoplasmic reticulum is responsible for transporting proteins through the cell. Lysosomes are small pouches in the cytoplasm that contain digestive enzymes. These vacuoles help the cell break down old or worn out organelles or cellular material.

20. C: Prokaryotes are single-celled organisms, which do not have nuclei. Their genetic material is condensed in the cytoplasm of the cell. Prokaryotes do have ribosomes and a cell membrane. Most also have a cell wall that aids in protection of the organism.

21. A: During metaphase, the chromosomes begin to line up in the center of the cell as the spindle fibers attach themselves to the centromeres on one end and the centrioles on the other. Next, anaphase occurs as the chromosomes are split into two identical sister chromatids. Prophase is the first stage of mitosis and refers to when the cell prepares for division: the nuclear membrane begins to break down, centrioles start migrating to the end of the cell, and the DNA becomes organized and prepared for mitosis. Telophase is the last stage of mitosis and occurs when the two chromatids start separating and the new nuclear envelopes begin to reform around the new nuclei.

22. B: There are four stages of Interphase:
1. G_1 (the stage immediately after the new daughter cells have been formed – the resting phase)

2. S (the stage of rapid DNA synthesis and replication),

3. G_2 (the stage of rapid cellular growth in preparation for mitosis), and

4. M (mitosis).

23. D: Meiosis is the process where one diploid (2n) cell will eventually divide to form four haploid (n) cells, which have half the number of chromosomes as the body cells. These haploid cells are gametes, not body cells.

24. D: The Krebs cycle actually occurs twice per molecule of glucose, as glucose is broken into two molecules of pyruvate, which are each eventually turned into acetyl-coA before entering the Krebs cycle. This cycle is an aerobic process, and it takes place in the inner part of the mitochondria.

25. C: The bulk of the energy released from ATP occurs when the first phosphate molecule breaks off AT to form ADP and phosphate. This is a hydrolysis reaction, meaning that it is facilitated by the water to break the bonds between phosphate and ADP. ATP is re-formed using a dehydration reaction, where water is removed from ADP and phosphate and they form a chemical bond.

ChemistryAnswer Key and Explanations

1. B: Mass is not the same as weight; rather, mass is the quantity of matter an object has.

2. C: There are three common states of matter: gases, liquids, and solids. The fourth state of matter, not commonly encountered on earth, is plasma.

3. D: An element is a substance that cannot be broken into simpler types of matter.

4. D: The two types of measurement important in science are quantitative (when a numerical result is used) and qualitative (when descriptions or qualities are reported).

5. D: A solid turns to a liquid by melting, and a liquid turns to a gas by vaporization.

6. B: An atom with an electrical charge is called an ion.

7. C: When atoms from two elements combine, the result is a molecule of a compound.

8. A: Freezing point is the point at which a liquid changes to a solid.

9. D: The rate at which a chemical reaction occurs does not depend on the amount of mass lost, since the law of conservation of mass (or matter) states that in a chemical reaction there is no loss of mass.

10. B: Boyle's law states that for a constant mass and temperature, pressure and volume are related inversely to one another: $PV = c$, where c = constant.

11. C: An ionic bond forms when one atom donates an electron from its outer shell, called a valence electron, to another atom to form two oppositely charged atoms.

12. B: Metals are usually solids at room temperature, while nonmetals are usually gases at room temperature.

13. D: A solution that contains more hydroxide ions than hydrogen ions is a base, and bases have a pH greater than 7, so the only possible answer is D, 9.

14. B: Magnesium oxide cannot be found on the periodic table because it is a compound of two elements.

15. C: A solute is a substance that is dissolved in another substance. In this case, the solute is the spices.

16. B: Coulomb's law describes the electric force between two charged particles. It states that like charges repel and opposite charges attract, and the greater their distance, the less force they will exert on each other.

17. C: Conduction is the transfer of thermal energy between two substances that come into contact with each other; their particles must collide in order to transfer energy.

18. A: Solids contain the least amount of kinetic energy because they are made up of closely packed atoms or molecules that are locked in position and exhibit very little movement. Gases and plasmas exhibit the greatest amount of energy.

19. C: Vectors have a magnitude (e.g., 5 meters/second) and direction (e.g., towards north). Of the choice listed, only velocity has a direction. (35 m/s north, for example). Speed, distance and time are all quantities that have a size but not a direction. That's why, for example, a car's speedometer reads 35 miles/hour, but does not indicate your direction of travel.

20. B: As you move from left to right across the periodic table, the atomic radius (size of the atom) decreases; it increases as you move down each group (from top to bottom). Electronegativity (the atom's ability to attract electrons), ionization energy (energy required to remove an electron from an atom), and electron affinity (the measure of energy changes with the addition of an electron) all generally increase as you move from left to right on the table. Moving down each group, electronegativity, ionization energy, and electron affinity all decrease.

21. A: Aluminum has a net charge of +3 (it's found in group 3 on the periodic table of elements). Hydroxide molecules are a group of atoms (hydrogen and oxygen) that have a net charge of -1. Therefore, you need three hydroxide groups are needed to balance the charge of the aluminum. The final molecular formula is $Al(OH)_3$.

22. D: According to Boyle's law, the pressure and volume of a gas are inversely related. The relationship between temperature and volume (they are directly related) is expressed in Charles' law. Avogadro's law describes how volume and the number of moles of a gas are related. PV = nRT is the ideal gas law and combines all of these variables in one master equation.

23. C: An alloy is a mixture of different elements and contains some of the properties of metals. Non-metals are found on the right side of the periodic table, while metals are found on the left. Network solids are exceptionally large and stable molecules with covalent bonds in multiple directions.

24. A: The process of sublimation occurs when a solid changes into a gas, while desublimation is the opposite process of changing a gas directly into a solid. Changing a liquid into a gas is called vaporization. Freezing is the name of the physical change from the liquid state to the solid state.

25. A: The pH of a solution is based on logarithmic relationships, specifically, powers of 10. This means that every point difference on the pH scale actually represents a tenfold change in the hydrogen ion concentration. If the pH decreases, the hydrogen ion concentration increases, and if the pH increases, hydrogen ion concentration decreases

Anatomy and Physiology Answer Key and Explanations

1.A: HCG is secreted by the trophoblast, part of the early embryo, following implantation in the uterus. GnRH (gonadotropin-releasing hormone. is secreted by the hypothalamus, while LH (luteinizing hormone. and FSH (follicle-stimulating hormone. are secreted by the pituitary gland. GnRH stimulates the production of LH and FSH. LH stimulates ovulation and the production of estrogen and progesterone by the ovary in females, and testosterone production in males. FSH stimulates maturation of the ovarian follicle and estrogen production in females and sperm production in males.

2. A: There are four basic tissue types in humans: epithelial, connective, nervous and muscular.

3. D: Skeletal, smooth, and cardiac are all types of muscle tissue. Adipose is not.

4. B: The only purpose of muscles is to produce movement through contraction

5. B: Anterior means toward the front of the body.

6. B: The brain is part of the nervous system.

7. B: Anatomy is the study of the structure and shape of the body.

8. A: Physiology is the study of how parts of the body function.

9. A: Circulation is transporting oxygen and other nutrients to the tissues via the cardiovascular system.

10. A: Smooth is not a type of connective tissue. Cartilage, adipose tissue, and blood tissue all are.

11. C: There are 11 organ systems in the human body.

12. B: The lymphatic system includes the spleen.

13. C: Proximal means close to the trunk of the body.

14. D: The lymphatic system, not the integumentary system, returns fluid to the blood vessels.

15. A: Optic refers to the eye or the way light is viewed.

16. A: Groups of cells that perform the same function are called tissues.

17. D: The nuclear division of somatic cells takes place during mitosis.

18. A: The immune system consists of the lymphatic system, spleen, tonsils, thymus and bone marrow.

19. A: A ribosome is a structure of eukaryotic cells that makes proteins.

20. A: Cortical bone is a connective tissue acting as a hard part of bones as organs. A liver is an organ, a mammal is a type of organism, and a hamstring is a muscle.

21. B: The adrenal glands are part of the endocrine system. They sit on the kidneys and produce hormones that regulate salt and water balance and influence blood pressure and heart rate.

22. B: Hemoglobin is a type of protein found in the red blood cells of all mammals.

23. D: Smooth muscle tissue involuntarily contracts to assist the digestive tract by moving the stomach and helping with the breakdown of food.

24. C: In respiration, food is used to produce energy as glucose and oxygen that react to produce carbon dioxide, water and ATP.

25. C: The pulmonary artery carries oxygen-depleted blood from the heart to the lungs, where CO_2 is released and the supply of oxygen is replenished. This blood then returns to the heart through the pulmonary vein, and is carried through the aorta and a series of branching arteries to the capillaries, where the bulk of gas exchange with the tissues occurs. Oxygen-depleted blood returns to the heart through branching veins (the femoral veins bring it from the legs) into the vena cava, which carries it again to the heart. Since the pulmonary artery is the last step before replenishment of the blood's oxygen content, it contains the blood which is the most oxygen depleted.

HESI A²PracticeTest #3

Reading Comprehension	Vocabulary and General Knowledge		Grammar		Mathematics	
1. ____	1. ____	49. ____	1. ____	49. ____	1. ____	49. ____
2. ____	2. ____	50. ____	2. ____	50. ____	2. ____	50. ____
3. ____	3. ____		3. ____		3. ____	
4. ____	4. ____		4. ____		4. ____	
5. ____	5. ____		5. ____		5. ____	
6. ____	6. ____		6. ____		6. ____	
7. ____	7. ____		7. ____		7. ____	
8. ____	8. ____		8. ____		8. ____	
9. ____	9. ____		9. ____		9. ____	
10. ____	10. ____		10. ____		10. ____	
11. ____	11. ____		11. ____		11. ____	
12. ____	12. ____		12. ____		12. ____	
13. ____	13. ____		13. ____		13. ____	
14. ____	14. ____		14. ____		14. ____	
15. ____	15. ____		15. ____		15. ____	
16. ____	16. ____		16. ____		16. ____	
17. ____	17. ____		17. ____		17. ____	
18. ____	18. ____		18. ____		18. ____	
19. ____	19. ____		19. ____		19. ____	
20. ____	20. ____		20. ____		20. ____	
21. ____	21. ____		21. ____		21. ____	
22. ____	22. ____		22. ____		22. ____	
23. ____	23. ____		23. ____		23. ____	
24. ____	24. ____		24. ____		24. ____	
25. ____	25. ____		25. ____		25. ____	
26. ____	26. ____		26. ____		26. ____	
27. ____	27. ____		27. ____		27. ____	
28. ____	28. ____		28. ____		28. ____	
29. ____	29. ____		29. ____		29. ____	
30. ____	30. ____		30. ____		30. ____	
31. ____	31. ____		31. ____		31. ____	
32. ____	32. ____		32. ____		32. ____	
33. ____	33. ____		33. ____		33. ____	
34. ____	34. ____		34. ____		34. ____	
35. ____	35. ____		35. ____		35. ____	
36. ____	36. ____		36. ____		36. ____	
37. ____	37. ____		37. ____		37. ____	
38. ____	38. ____		38. ____		38. ____	
39. ____	39. ____		39. ____		39. ____	
40. ____	40. ____		40. ____		40. ____	
41. ____	41. ____		41. ____		41. ____	
42. ____	42. ____		42. ____		42. ____	
43. ____	43. ____		43. ____		43. ____	
44. ____	44. ____		44. ____		44. ____	
45. ____	45. ____		45. ____		45. ____	
46. ____	46. ____		46. ____		46. ____	
47. ____	47. ____		47. ____		47. ____	
	48. ____		48. ____		48. ____	

Biology	Chemistry	Anatomy and Physiology
1. _____	1. _____	1. _____
2. _____	2. _____	2. _____
3. _____	3. _____	3. _____
4. _____	4. _____	4. _____
5. _____	5. _____	5. _____
6. _____	6. _____	6. _____
7. _____	7. _____	7. _____
8. _____	8. _____	8. _____
9. _____	9. _____	9. _____
10. _____	10. _____	10. _____
11. _____	11. _____	11. _____
12. _____	12. _____	12. _____
13. _____	13. _____	13. _____
14. _____	14. _____	14. _____
15. _____	15. _____	15. _____
16. _____	16. _____	16. _____
17. _____	17. _____	17. _____
18. _____	18. _____	18. _____
19. _____	19. _____	19. _____
20. _____	20. _____	20. _____
21. _____	21. _____	21. _____
22. _____	22. _____	22. _____
23. _____	23. _____	23. _____
24. _____	24. _____	24. _____
25. _____	25. _____	25. _____

Section 1. Reading Comprehension

Number of Questions: **47**
Time Limit: **50 Minutes**

Questions 1–10 pertain to the following passage:

The disease known as rickets causes the bones to soften and creates a risk of bone fractures and even permanent bone deformation. It is most common in children, since their bones are already soft and are still growing. Rickets is believed to result from a lack of vitamin D and calcium, although some researchers will add a lack of phosphorus to this list. The disease is usually seen in parts of the world where children are suffering from poor nutrition. In the United States, doctors believed that the disease has been all but obsolete since the end of the Great Depression.

In fact, they were mistaken. Doctors are seeing a return of rickets, not just in the United States but also in other places where it was long since written off as no longer something to worry about. Cases of rickets are on the rise in states such as Georgia and North Carolina, and doctors are not entirely sure of the cause. They attribute the likely cause of the condition to poor nutrition and a lack of necessary vitamins and minerals. Many doctors believe that there is a twofold problem: low levels of calcium in young children who do not consume enough dairy products and low levels of vitamin D in breastfed babies. While breastfeeding is recommended, doctors point out that breast milk does not naturally contain high levels of vitamin D. This can be fine if the mother herself has adequate levels, but mothers with low levels of vitamin D will not provide enough for the baby as it nurses.

Among other developed nations, rickets is also making a reappearance in Great Britain. Doctors across England are seeing unexpected cases of rickets in children, and they believe that this is connected largely to low vitamin D levels. Some blame is placed on weather conditions, since Great Britain is not known for having copious amounts of sunshine, but also on lifestyle. Children are spending more time indoors watching television and playing video games, and in doing so they miss the sunshine when it is available. Additionally parents are having their children wear sunscreen, which appears to be blocking what vitamin D would be absorbed while the children are outdoors.

Rickets is not yet considered an epidemic in developed nations, but there is enough concern among doctors and researchers to encourage awareness among parents. Children are encouraged to spend some time outdoors and to allow their skin to receive a little sun—just a few minutes a day is enough. Vitamin D and calcium supplements are also recommended, and nursing mothers are advised to have their levels checked. With any luck, rickets will once again become a disease of the past.

1. What is the author's primary purpose in writing the essay?
   A. to persuade
   B. to inform
   C. to analyze
   D. to entertain

2. What is the main idea of the passage?
    A. Rickets should once again be a disease of the past
    B. Rickets has once again become a problem in some developed nations
    C. Children need vitamin D and calcium to avoid rickets, and nursing mothers need to have their levels checked
    D. Rickets has reappeared only in the United States and Great Britain

3. Which of the following is *not* a detail from the passage?
    A. A lack of phosphorus is a possible contributor to rickets
    B. Sunscreen can block the skin's absorption of necessary vitamin D
    C. Adults in Great Britain also have low vitamin D levels
    D. Rickets has not been a problem in the United States since the time after the Great Depression

4. Based on the information provided in the passage, what can the reader infer about why the return of rickets is such a surprise in the United States?
    A. The diet in the United States has improved since the Great Depression
    B. People are already taking vitamin D and calcium supplements
    C. Unlike in Great Britain, there is plenty of sunshine in many parts of the United States
    D. Children in the United States spend enough time playing outdoors without wearing sunscreen

5. Which of the following *cannot* be inferred from the information in the passage?
    A. Rickets has always been most common in third world nations among people who have a poor diet
    B. Nursing mothers with low vitamin D levels should consider adding a supplement to their diet
    C. The number of rickets cases in developed nations is not necessarily high, but the rise in expected cases is enough to concern doctors about the cause
    D. Doctors are advising mothers with nursing babies to use formula that supplements vitamin D

6. Which of the following *can* be inferred from the information in the passage?
    A. Doctors believe that the cases of rickets in Great Britain are linked more to lack of vitamin D than to low levels of calcium
    B. Doctors now believe that children should not wear sunscreen while playing outside
    C. Nursing mothers in Great Britain typically have higher levels of vitamin D in their breast milk
    D. The majority of researchers believe that rickets is caused by lack of vitamin D and calcium only

7. The author uses the term *developed nations* to indicate which of the following in the passage?
    A. nations that are constantly improving the status quo for citizens
    B. nations that are world leaders in politics and economics
    C. nations in which citizens receive plenty of sunshine for vitamin D absorption
    D. nations in which most citizens have access to adequate nutritional options

8. What is the meaning of the word *copious* as it is used in the third paragraph?
    A. abundant
    B. small
    C. expected
    D. appropriate

9. What is the purpose of the final paragraph of the passage?
   A. to offer solutions for preventing and eliminating rickets
   B. to advise developing nations on how to avoid rickets
   C. to warn nursing mothers about the importance of vitamin D
   D. to provide hope for the future of a world without rickets

10. Which of the following is *not* a recommendation for ridding developed nations of rickets, as presented by the author?
   A. People should consider taking vitamin D and calcium supplements
   B. Children should get a little sun each day
   C. Television and video games should be limited among children
   D. Nursing mothers should have their vitamin D and calcium levels checked

Questions 11–20 pertain to the following passage:

So your children got the chicken pox vaccine, and you think they will be all right. Not so fast. As it turns out, the chicken pox vaccine may only increase the risk of problems over time. Make no mistake: vaccination is not necessarily a bad thing, and vaccines have gone a long way toward eliminating illnesses that were once feared as life threatening or permanently disabling. But vaccines for some diseases, chicken pox in particular, come with side effects that create long-term uneasiness for doctors and researchers.

In fact, many scientists are increasingly concerned that *not* getting chicken pox might be more dangerous. Many people remember chicken pox as a standard childhood disease. Everyone seemed to get it, and everyone who had it probably knows that it is supposed to be a one-time deal. In others words, you catch chicken pox, scratch for about a week, and you never see it again—at least in theory. What happens in reality is that once a person catches chicken pox, the virus stays in the body. It typically remains dormant for the life of the individual, however, and the reason for this is only now being appreciated.

Researchers believe that those who have had chicken pox, those with the dormant virus in their bodies, should be around others who have had the disease. Doing so actually appears to boost the body's ongoing immunity against the virus. This means that spending time around children who have or have had chicken pox can help ensure that it never comes back. It can also help prevent the disease known as shingles later in life. Shingles, which is a more severe version of chicken pox, usually strikes adults after the age of sixty and can come with far more severe side effects than one week of scratching and sitting in an oatmeal bath. In some cases, shingles can cause problems that affect the sufferer for the rest of his or her life. But there appears to be a natural immunity that is built into getting chicken pox and then being around others with chicken pox, and researchers now believe that this explains the low rate of shingles that has traditionally been seen in the United States.

But what happens if very few people get chicken pox and most people are vaccinated? Children who are vaccinated do not contract the disease, and the amount of virus in the vaccine is not enough to boost immunity and thus prevent the contraction of shingles in many adults. And shingles is particularly dangerous because many of the elderly who contract it are already in poor health and struggle to recover from it. Some epidemiologists suggest that the use of the chicken pox vaccine in the United States alone could lead to more than 20 million cases of shingles and at least 5,000 deaths from the disease. The potential concerns scientists enough that there remains ongoing debate about the value of the chicken pox vaccine.

11. What is the main idea of the passage?
   A. Getting the chicken pox vaccine can lead to shingles later in life
   B. Many children are getting the chicken pox vaccine throughout the United States
   C. The chicken pox vaccine has the potential to create long-term problems
   D. Chickenpox is no longer a childhood disease, as many adults now contract it

12. What is the author's primary purpose in writing the essay?
   A. to entertain
   B. to persuade
   C. to analyze
   D. to inform

13. Based on the information in the passage, what does an *epidemiologist* do?
   A. study diseases among a population
   B. study the internal organs of the human body
   C. study viruses that are contracted among children
   D. study adult problems that develop from childhood diseases

14. Which of the following is *not* a detail from the passage?
   A. There are deaths from chicken pox each year in the United States
   B. Shingles is a disease that develops from the same virus as chicken pox
   C. Some researchers believe that not getting chicken pox can cause problems
   D. Adults who contract shingles face a more dangerous disease than chicken pox

15. Based on the information in the passage, what is the value in contracting chicken pox during childhood?
   A. to get it over with as early as possible
   B. to avoid contracting shingles later in life
   C. to have the dormant virus in the body throughout life
   D. to demonstrate the body's natural immunity to some viruses

16. Based on the information in the passage, why is it important for people who have had chicken pox to be around others who have or have had the disease?
   A. to help keep the disease in circulation and avoid shingles
   B. to keep from catching chicken pox again
   C. to boost the body's immunity to the virus
   D. to maintain a low level of adult-contracted shingles

17. Which of the following *cannot* be inferred from the information in the passage?
   A. People typically have contracted chicken pox in childhood
   B. The age of shingles sufferers contributes to its serious effects on health
   C. Many vaccines have helped rid society of dangerous diseases
   D. Researchers believe that no one should get the chicken pox vaccine

18. Based on the information in the passage, why are some scientists concerned about extensive vaccination against chicken pox?
    A. There is very little disease in the vaccine, but it is just enough for adults who have not had chicken pox to contract shingles
    B. Researchers will be unable to locate enough subjects for ongoing study of health patterns among those who contract the disease
    C. The contraction of chicken pox among adults is far more inconvenient than it is for children, so it is easier to contract the disease in childhood
    D. Without frequent outbreaks of the disease, those who have already had it cannot build up their immunity to it

19. Which of the following pieces of information would make the author's point about the projected cases of shingles and deaths from shingles stronger in the final paragraph?
    A. the names of researchers who are active in educating people about the chicken pox vaccine
    B. the time period for the projected cases of shingles and the deaths from shingles
    C. the countries where the chicken pox vaccine is currently in wide use
    D. the number of people who are vaccinated against chicken pox each year

20. Which of the following *can* be inferred from the information in the final sentence?
    A. More and more researchers are advising against widespread vaccination against chicken pox
    B. The numbers are enough to concern researchers that the chicken pox vaccine might prove to do more harm than good
    C. Researchers continue to evaluate and consider the long-term effects of the chicken pox vaccine
    D. The concern about the effects of the chicken pox vaccine has led to a decrease in vaccinations

Questions 21–30 pertain to the following passage:

It seems like an obvious choice: do we destroy the final remaining samples of the smallpox virus or not? Smallpox, the terror that ravaged nations for centuries, was virtually destroyed in the latter part of the twentieth century—but not before it took about 500,000,000 people with it. Smallpox is one of the most dangerous viruses, attacking only humans (but not animals) and leaving only 70 percent of those infected with it alive. In some cases, survival brought its own challenges. The virus has been known to leave severe scarring, and many victims also lost their eyesight. Smallpox is so virulent that the small amount in the vaccine has been known to cause minor side effects.

So why would anyone want to keep samples around? Why not destroy what is left of the disease and eradicate it for good? After its successful inoculation program, the World Health Organization (WHO) has continued to maintain a selection of smallpox virus samples; more than 400 samples sit in laboratories in the United States and in Russia. The WHO has agreed that the samples should be consigned to the dustbin of history. They just cannot agree on whether all samples should be destroyed, and when the destruction should occur. The Soviet Union collapsed in 1991, but there were suggestions that the Soviet government, among others, had hidden samples of the smallpox virus separate from the official samples that were acknowledged. Should the WHO destroy all official samples, any remaining unofficial samples (never confirmed to be real) could be used to attack a population in an act of bioterrorism. Without its own samples, the WHO and its researchers might be unable to create an effective treatment or vaccine.

Bioterrorism remains a real threat, and smallpox continues to be a concern for those looking at potential diseases that terrorists might use. What is more, the WHO points out that the majority of people today have no defense against outbreaks of the disease. Inoculation against smallpox ended in the early 1980s, and smallpox was declared to be officially defeated. Should a terrorist chose to attack people with smallpox, most would be completely susceptible to its dangers. As a result, many scientists—and particularly those who study infectious diseases—believe that the WHO should continue to delay destruction of the smallpox virus samples. Others claim that there are currently effective vaccines that could be used to protect a population. Even the two nations that hold these final samples are at loggerheads about the issue. One thing seems to be certain: the WHO still agrees that the smallpox samples should be destroyed. They just do not seem to know how *many* of the samples to destroy and *how soon*.

21. Which of the following words describes the author's primary purpose in writing the essay?
   A. persuasive
   B. Investigative
   C. Expository
   D. Advisory

22. What is the main idea of the passage?
   A. The smallpox vaccine should be destroyed to eradicate the disease and prevent future outbreaks
   B. The smallpox vaccine should not be destroyed to maintain samples that can be used in the event of a bioterrorism attack
   C. The United States and Russia cannot agree on how many of the remaining smallpox samples to destroy, so the World Health Organization has stepped in to assist
   D. The World Health Organization would prefer to destroy remaining samples of the smallpox vaccine but cannot decide when to do so

23. Which of the following is *not* a detail from the passage?
   A. Smallpox killed at least half a billion people in the twentieth century alone
   B. Samples of the smallpox virus are still kept in the Soviet Union
   C. The smallpox virus has been known to cause both scarring and blindness
   D. The World Health Organization instituted a smallpox vaccination program to eradicate the disease

24. Based on the information in the passage, what does the word *consigned* mean?
   A. sent
   B. refused
   C. kept
   D. hidden

25. Based on the information in the passage, why might the World Health Organization want to retain samples of the smallpox virus?
   A. to develop a treatment and vaccine in the event of bioterrorism
   B. to prevent acts of bioterrorism from those who hold secret samples of smallpox
   C. to utilize the samples for continued research on the smallpox virus
   D. to institute a new vaccination program that will protect people against future acts of bioterrorism

26. Which of the following *cannot* be inferred from the information in the passage?
    A. The majority of people who contract the smallpox virus survive
    B. The members of the World Health Organization are still trying to decide if all of the smallpox virus samples should be destroyed
    C. The smallpox virus is one of the diseases that create concerns of bioterrorism for the World Health Organization
    D. The World Health Organization is confident that there are secret samples of the smallpox virus being stored by terrorists

27. Based on the information in the passage, why do some researchers believe that it is now safe to destroy the remaining samples of the smallpox virus?
    A. Because the disease is essentially obsolete, there is no need to maintain samples of it against future outbreaks
    B. The collapse of the Soviet Union removed the risk of bioterrorism from the samples stored in that country and the United States
    C. There is already a smallpox vaccine that could be used to protect people against outbreaks of the disease
    D. Enough people have already been vaccinated against the smallpox virus and are protected against acts of bioterrorism

28. Since the World Health Organization was responsible for an inoculation program against smallpox, what can be inferred about the WHO's concern that the majority of people today are susceptible to the virus?
    A. There are not enough people who are choosing to be vaccinated against smallpox
    B. Very few are vaccinated today, and the vaccine has worn off for those who did receive it in the 1980s
    C. The risks that accompany the smallpox vaccine have created concerns and have resulted in a reduction of vaccinations
    D. Since smallpox is no longer seen as a threat, the majority of people do not believe that they are in any danger of contracting the virus

29. Based on the context of the passage, which of the following is the best definition for the expression *at loggerheads* in the final paragraph?
    A. considering options
    B. quietly discussing
    C. eager to decide
    D. in disagreement

30. Which of the following is *not* a detail from the passage?
    A. The World Health Organization developed a widespread vaccination program and successfully combated the smallpox virus
    B. While once considered a disease that only humans could contract, smallpox is slowly beginning to infect animals as well
    C. Smallpox has been known to cause blindness in those who survive the disease
    D. There are concerns that unofficial samples of the smallpox vaccine might have made it into the hands of governments other than that of the Soviet Union

Questions 31–37 pertain to the following passage:

The Black Death, a rapid and widespread outbreak of plague, first struck Europe in the fourteenth century. It also made several brief reappearances over the following centuries until it finally died off in the nineteenth century. Historians believe that the plague was responsible for the deaths of more than 50 percent of the population, killing between 75 million and 100 million people. The greatest fear of the Black Death was the sense of the unknown that it brought with it. The disease struck and spread quickly, and medieval doctors had no idea what caused it. (Today, many believe that rats were responsible for spreading the fleas that carried the disease. Oddly enough, many medieval people believed that it was the cats that were responsible and killed a large number of them, thus decreasing the opportunity to remove the real culprits.) Additionally, the plague killed some and not others—for no clear reason—and there was no known cure. Between 90 percent and 95 percent of those who contracted the disease died, and most within a week.

To understand the cause of such a devastating epidemic, scientists and historians have had to look back into history and piece together a puzzle. The majority accept the theory of the bubonic plague: rats carrying infected fleas made their way to various parts of Europe after arriving in the port cities, where the disease struck first. Some are not so sure, however. A few have argued that the flea-and-rat theory does not fit in with the symptoms, since fleas tend to attack the lower parts of the body, and it was the upper lymph nodes that showed the worse inflammation. Others point out that it would have been difficult for the fleas to stay alive long enough to infect people and spread the disease in Europe's cooler climate. One theory points to anthrax from cattle as a possible culprit, while another sees similarities between the spread of the Black Death and the spread of the Ebola virus. The exact cause(s) might never be known for certain. What is certain, though, is that the Black Death permanently changed Europe—and that no one wants to see it return.

31. Which of the following best describes the author's tone in the passage?
    A. playful
    B. concerned
    C. definitive
    D. explanatory

32. What is the main idea in the passage?
    A. The Black Death had devastating effects in Europe, but scientists and historians are still not certain about what caused it
    B. The spread of the Black Death suggests that the traditional theory about rats carrying infected fleas might not be accurate
    C. The Black Death could have been prevented if medieval people had kept their cats alive instead of killing them
    D. The Black Death was responsible for destroying more than half of Europe's population and is believed to have killed 100 million people

33. Which of the following is *not* a detail from the passage?
    A. Europe continued to see outbreaks of the Black Death until the nineteenth century
    B. Some scientists and historians have disagreed with the traditional view that infected fleas caused the Black Death
    C. In addition to striking much of Europe, the Black Death also spread into parts of Asia
    D. Medieval doctors were unsure of what caused the Black Death and could not treat it effectively

34. Which of the following *cannot* be inferred from the passage?
    A. There might be more than one cause of the Black Death
    B. The infection that caused the Black Death is related to the Ebola virus
    C. While the death rate was high, some people survived the Black Death
    D. The Black Death had far-reaching effects in Europe

35. Based on the information in the passage, why do some scientists and historians question the theory about the bubonic plague?
    A. The symptoms of the Black Death and the climate of Europe appear to contradict the theory
    B. The victims of the Black Death should have experienced inflammation in their lower lymph nodes
    C. Current research suggests that the infection resembles anthrax more than bubonic plague
    D. The fleas carrying the infection could not have lived long enough to create such a widespread epidemic

36. In the first paragraph, why does the author use parentheses around two of the sentences?
    A. to create emphasis for the reader and indicate where the most important points are
    B. to strengthen the main point by presenting important historical detail
    C. to indicate interesting information that does not fit within the primary flow of thought
    D. to include a supporting example from another source

37. Based on the information in the passage, which of the following can be assumed?
    A. It is impossible to know for sure what caused the Black Death
    B. The Ebola virus tends to spread quickly, just like the Black Death
    C. Modern medicine has ensured that there will be no further outbreaks of the Black Death
    D. Medieval doctors applied superstitious methods to treat outbreaks of the Black Death

Questions 38–42 pertain to the following passage:

It is a common summer ailment, and one that sends more than two million people to the doctor annually. It also tends to be a condition that most people forget about, until it is too late of course. Swimmer's ear might seem like a simple enough problem—a little water in the ear, a bit of swelling for a few days, some itching—but it affects millions of Americans annually and costs the medical industry at least $500 million per year. It can also create problems well beyond a few days of inconvenience. That is a lot for just a little water in the ear.

The problem, of course, is not the water itself but rather the quality of it and what happens when it remains in the ear canal. Swimming pools fill up during the summer months, and even the chlorine cannot keep the bacteria out. The bacteria that ends up floating in the water alongside swimmers can get into the ear canal, and when it does an infection can develop. Officially, this infection is known as otitis externa, but anyone who has experienced it knows it simply as swimmer's ear. With swimmer's ear, the ear canal becomes inflamed and, in extreme cases, can spread to the outside of the ear and even to parts of the face. In some, swimmer's ear has been known to cause temporary hearing loss.

The key to avoiding this condition is protecting the ears while around water and getting any water out as soon as possible. The longer that water remains in the ear canal, the better the chances that the bacteria will take up residence and cause an infection. If there is water in the ear, people are advised to avoid the old "head-banging" routine and utilize alcohol instead, as this pulls water out effectively without rattling the brain around. Doctors also advise using a soft towel to draw the water out, and some suggest using a blow dryer to remove the water.

38. What are the author's primary purposes in writing the essay?
    A. to define and expand
    B. to inform and advise
    C. to present and persuade
    D. to explain and approve

39. Which of the following *cannot* be inferred from the information in the passage?
    A. Water in swimming pools can contain bacteria that causes infections in the ear canal
    B. The infection that causes swimmer's ear leads to swelling in the ear canal
    C. Swimmer's ear starts as a simple infection but can cause more serious problems
    D. Anyone who gets water in his or her ear can expect to develop swimmer's ear

40. Which of the following is *not* a detail from the passage?
    A. People can develop swimmer's ear from being in any body of water during the summer
    B. The medical name for swimmer's ear is otitis externa
    C. Swimmer's ear affects over one million people in the United States each year
    D. Swimmer's ear results from bacteria in the water that gets into people's ear canals

41. Based on the information in the passage, why is swimmer's ear such a problem for people who spend time in swimming pools in the summer?
    A. People shed body oils, skin, and bacteria when they use swimming pools, and these are a breeding ground for disease
    B. Swimming pool maintenance crews cannot keep up with the increased activity in the pool during the hot summer months
    C. The chlorine in the water is not sufficient to destroy the bacteria from such a large number of people in the pool
    D. Swimmers do not use earplugs as much as they should, and this provides an opportunity for bacteria to get into the ear canal

42. Based on the information in the passage, which of the following is *not* a recommended course of action for removing water from the ear canal?
    A. using alcohol to draw the water out
    B. pressing a towel against the ear
    C. shaking the head vigorously
    D. drying the water with a blow dryer

Questions 43–47 pertain to the following passage:
It struck almost without warning: a headache, a chill, aching joints. A few hours later, the heat set in, and this led to intense sweating, dehydration, and delirium. Within a few more hours, death was expected to follow. The English of the fifteenth and sixteenth centuries were not sure what this disease was or what caused it; they only knew it as the "sweating sickness." Tens of thousands fell prey to it, and even though the numbers are not as high as some epidemics, the fear of the sweating sickness was greater due to the mystery surrounding it. Even today, the disease, not to mention its origin, has still not been identified. The sweating sickness disappeared from England in the 1570s, but the fact that no one is sure of what caused it leaves the door open for a possible return at some point.

Hygiene and sanitation are always the first culprits when searching for the source of an epidemic. Evils such as typhus and cholera are typically linked to filthy conditions in which disease can develop and spread. In general, these diseases tend to erupt first among the economically depressed who live in squalid conditions. But in the case of the sweating sickness, the disease seemed to have a magnetic attraction to the upper classes instead of the poor, and if anyone was more likely to be clean and have adequate sanitation, it was the wealthy.

Some scientists have suggested a bacterial fever, but the most likely results from the bites of lice and ticks. The English doctors who wrote about the disease made no mention of seeing such signs on victims. The latest theory points to the possibility of a hantavirus, which is a fast-acting disease that is carried by rodents and passed on when humans come in contact with them or their waste (however unintentionally). In the England of the fifteenth and sixteenth centuries, rodents were certainly a problem for rich and poor alike. But the problem with this theory is that humans cannot spread a hantavirus—as far as scientists know—but they almost certainly spread the sweating sickness. The cause of the sweating sickness might remain shrouded in mystery for now, but doctors and scientists continue research to make sure another epidemic does not occur in the future.

43. What is the main idea of the passage?
   A. The sweating sickness was a mysterious illness that broke out in England in the fifteenth and sixteenth centuries, and scientists are still unsure about what caused it
   B. The cause of the sweating sickness mystified fifteenth and sixteenth century doctors, but scientists today are beginning to solve the mystery of what caused the disease
   C. The sweating sickness briefly attacked England in the fifteenth and sixteenth centuries, and it has not broken out anywhere since then
   D. Modern-day scientists have narrowed the causes of sweating sickness down to a few options, but the lack of reporting from the fifteenth and sixteenth centuries make it impossible to confirm the cause

44. Which of the following is *not* a detail from the passage?
   A. The sweating sickness struck quickly and often killed victims within a few hours
   B. The sweating sickness is believed to have been caused by human contact with rodents and their waste
   C. Doctors in the fifteenth and sixteenth centuries did not notice any strange bites that would suggest lice or ticks spread the sweating sickness
   D. No cases of the sweating sickness have been seen in England since the latter part of the sixteenth century

45. Based on the information in the passage, which of the following can be inferred?
   A. The sweating sickness was more likely to strike the wealthy instead of the poor in fifteenth and sixteenth century England
   B. The sweating sickness is believed to have been spread from human contact
   C. Other epidemics in England have resulted in far more deaths than the sweating sickness
   D. The sweating sickness does not appear to have been caused by bad hygiene and sanitation among the poor

46. Based on the information in the passage, which of the following is known about hantaviruses?
   A. Hantaviruses result from poor sanitary conditions and bad hygiene among the lower classes
   B. Hantaviruses are carried by rodents and spread to humans through contact with rodents
   C. Scientists now believe that some hantaviruses can be spread from contact between humans
   D. The symptoms of the sweating sickness indicate that a hantavirus was the most likely cause

47. Based on the information in the passage, which of the following can be inferred about the sweating sickness?
    A. Modern medical treatments mean that a return of the sweating sickness would not cause the same problems as it did in fifteenth and sixteenth century England
    B. Doctors in fifteenth and sixteenth century England lacked the observational skills to notice any signs of bites from lice and ticks on patients
    C. Because they do not know the cause, doctors and scientists are unsure about whether a new epidemic of sweating sickness will occur
    D. The relatively low number of deaths from the sweating sickness suggests that many people in fifteenth and sixteenth century England did survive the disease

Section 2. Vocabulary and General Knowledge

Number of Questions: **50**	
Time Limit: **50 Minutes**	

1. What is the meaning of the word *bifurcate*?
   A. close
   B. glow
   C. split
   D. speak

2. What is the best definition for the word *influx*?
   A. acceptance
   B. complexity
   C. arrival
   D. theory

3. What is the meaning of the word *substantiate*?
   A. inhibit
   B. assume
   C. confirm
   D. complete

4. What is the best definition for the word *typify*?
   A. obscure
   B. mock
   C. announce
   D. symbolize

5. What is the best definition for the word *sinuous*?
   A. ominous
   B. spoiled
   C. supple
   D. elaborate

6. What is the best definition for the word *insidious*?
   A. loyal
   B. subtle
   C. intelligent
   D. unlikely

7. What is the best definition for the word *emaciated*?
   A. vivid
   B. fresh
   C. grateful
   D. wasted

8. What is the meaning of the word *irrevocable*?
   A. binding
   B. fortunate
   C. unfeasible
   D. indefinite

9. What is the meaning of the word *abate*?
   A. enhance
   B. remove
   C. revive
   D. reduce

10. What is the best definition for the word *extirpate*?
   A. assist
   B. define
   C. provide
   D. remove

11. What is the meaning of the word *feckless*?
   A. incompetent
   B. significant
   C. relevant
   D. headstrong

12. What is the meaning of the word *constrict*?
   A. collect
   B. appreciate
   C. tighten
   D. mingle

13. What is the meaning of the word *goad*?
   A. create
   B. force
   C. bore
   D. please

14. Select the meaning of the underlined word in this sentence:
With so much uncertainty about which decision was the best, the school provost submitted the various proposals to the board and ultimately chose the most <u>prevalent</u> favorite among the members.
   A. dominant
   B. old-fashioned
   C. indifferent
   D. scarce

15. What is the meaning of the word *nonchalant*?
   A. excited
   B. cowardly
   C. unconcerned
   D. imprudent

16. What is the best definition for the word *malinger*?
    A. meet
    B. prevent
    C. pretend
    D. surge

17. What is the meaning of the word *serrated*?
    A. unusual
    B. defiant
    C. sad
    D. jagged

18. What is the meaning of the word *contiguous*?
    A. unique
    B. adjacent
    C. indirect
    D. pleased

19. What is the meaning of the word *obfuscate*?
    A. resemble
    B. decide
    C. conceal
    D. surpass

20. What is the best definition for the word *portend*?
    A. withdraw
    B. deny
    C. uncover
    D. forecast

21. Select the best definition for the underlined word in this sentence:
Although Nina was disappointed by the rude comment her supervisor made at the staff meeting, she decided to speak to him privately so he did not think she was trying to underline him in front of everyone else.
    A. disturb
    B. encourage
    C. challenge
    D. present

22. What is the meaning of the word *immutable*?
    A. unchangeable
    B. breakable
    C. desirable
    D. flexible

23. What is the best definition for the word *protracted*?
    A. required
    B. extended
    C. elevated
    D. delayed

24. What is the best definition for the word *viable*?
    A. inanimate
    B. reasonable
    C. likely
    D. living

25. What is the best definition for the word *incessant*?
    A. complicated
    B. uncertain
    C. constant
    D. frightening

26. What is the meaning of the word *negligible*?
    A. adequate
    B. significant
    C. minor
    D. careless

27. What is the meaning of the word *accost*?
    A. confront
    B. insult
    C. mock
    D. evade

28. What is the meaning of the word *retreat*?
    A. provide
    B. contain
    C. withdraw
    D. anger

29. What is the meaning of the word *dichotomy*?
    A. formation
    B. decision
    C. interruption
    D. split

30. What is the best definition for the word *solicitous*?
    A. plentiful
    B. attentive
    C. ignorant
    D. stubborn

31. What is the best definition for the word *trajectory*?
    A. direction
    B. excitement
    C. simplification
    D. calculation

32. Select the meaning of the underlined word in this sentence:
The teacher took Agnes to task for her <u>unwarranted</u> comment about the new students in the class and how they were unable to afford better clothes.
  A. justifiable
  B. biased
  C. essential
  D. inappropriate

33. What is the meaning of the word *intemperate*?
  A. unrestrained
  B. unconcerned
  C. idle
  D. organized

34. What is the meaning of the word *onerous*?
  A. trivial
  B. motivating
  C. demanding
  D. urgent

35. What is the meaning of the word *heterogeneous*?
  A. different
  B. unusual
  C. clear
  D. comparable

36. What is the best definition for the word *overwrought*?
  A. agitated
  B. respected
  C. indifferent
  D. excessive

37. What is the best definition for the word *dotage*?
  A. strength
  B. senility
  C. balance
  D. position

38. What is the best definition for the word *puerile*?
  A. youthful
  B. sophisticated
  C. virtuous
  D. childish

39. What is the meaning of the word *putative*?
  A. chosen
  B. factual
  C. accepted
  D. affective

40. What is the meaning of the word *enumerate*?
    A. refuse
    B. plead
    C. include
    D. specify

41. What is the best definition for the word *intangible*?
    A. sudden
    B. vague
    C. forthright
    D. definite

42. What is the meaning of the word *relapse*?
    A. prevention
    B. endearment
    C. progression
    D. setback

43. What is the best definition for the word *definitive*?
    A. absurd
    B. incomplete
    C. ultimate
    D. preferred

44. What is the meaning of the word *conflate*?
    A. falsify
    B. merge
    C. anticipate
    D. expand

45. What is the best definition for the word *congenital*?
    A. contracted
    B. lifelong
    C. additional
    D. innate

46. What is the best definition for the word *gestate*?
    A. conceive
    B. provide
    C. delete
    D. remind

47. What is the meaning of the word *mordant*?
    A. elegant
    B. soothing
    C. joking
    D. disrespectful

48. What is the meaning of the word *transmute*?
    A. annoy
    B. maintain
    C. change
    D. charge

49. What is the meaning of the word *circumscribe*?
    A. continue
    B. enclose
    C. converse
    D. permit

50. What is the best definition for the word *prehensile*?
    A. gentle
    B. clever
    C. greedy
    D. gracious

Section 3. Grammar

| Number of Questions: **50** |
| Time Limit: **50 Minutes** |

1. Select the combination of words that makes the following sentence grammatically correct. Detective Melchior tried to _____ the solution by winking vigorously, but his sidekick was unable to _____ the detective's meaning and asked, "Why are you winking, sir?"
    A. infer, imply
    B. imply, infer
    C. imply, imply
    D. infer, infer

2. Select the following sentence that is in the *active tense*.
    A. The child was given presents by his friends for his birthday
    B. The winner of the marathon was rewarded with a medal by the awards committee
    C. The fashion designer presented his newest collection on the Paris runways
    D. The aromatic duck a l'orange was quickly devoured by the eager culinary students

3. Select the combination of words that makes the following sentence grammatically correct. _____ of my time is spent in completing the _____ tasks that I have each day.
    A. many, much
    B. many, many
    C. much, many
    D. much, much

4. Select the combination of words that makes the following sentence grammatically correct. Because Edwina had _____ time than she expected, she ran to the express lane in the grocery store, despite the fact that she had more than the required "Ten Items or _____."
    A. fewer, fewer
    B. fewer, less
    C. less, less
    D. less, fewer

5. Select the word or phrase that is correctly capitalized for the following sentence. The eighth-grade students recently completed their study of the Battle of Verdun during _____.
    A. world war I
    B. World War I
    C. World war i
    D. World war I

6. Select the word or phrase that is correctly capitalized for the following sentence. Historians have traditionally believed that more than one million people died during the _____, but some argue that the figure should be revised to upward of four million.
    A. siege of Leningrad
    B. siege Of Leningrad
    C. Siege of Leningrad
    D. siege of leningrad

7. Select the word or phrase that is correctly capitalized for the following sentence.
Leo's planetary studies led him to review Saturn, Neptune, Jupiter, _____.
   A. Earth, and the Sun
   B. earth, and the Sun
   C. Earth, and the sun
   D. earth, and the sun

8. Select the word or phrase that is correctly abbreviated for the following sentence.
The doctor wrote out the details of the prescription, noting the specific amount of milligrams that the patient needed to take: "_____ to be taken each day."
   A. 4 mlg
   B. 4 mgr
   C. 4 m
   D. 4 mg

9. Select the word or phrase that makes the following sentence grammatically correct.
My two friends, Janet and _____, are planning to join us at the opera this weekend.
   A. she
   B. her
   C. they
   D. them

10. Select the word or phrase that makes the following sentence grammatically correct.
Emily noticed that the book was not sitting where she had left it, and she shrieked, "Somebody _____ been in my house!"
   A. have
   B. will
   C. has
   D. might

11. Select the word or phrase that makes the following sentence grammatically correct.
The head of the student council noted, "With the increase in tuition prices, the financial burden placed on _____ guarantees that we will be expected to pay far more than we can reasonably afford."
   A. those students
   B. we students
   C. us students
   D. them students

12. Select the word or phrase that makes the following sentence grammatically correct.
The new benefit plan applies to _____ employees in the agency.
   A. part- and full-time
   B. part and full-time
   C. part and full time
   D. part/ and full/time

13. Select the combination of words that makes the following sentence grammatically correct.
_____ that foul-smelling cup of tea away, and _____ me something that I can actually drink.
   A. bring, take
   B. bring, bring
   C. take, bring
   D. take, take

14. Select the word or phrase that makes the following sentence grammatically correct.
You _____ to get your oil changed before you damage your vehicle.
    A. ought
    B. had ought
    C. should ought
    D. had

15. Select the word or phrase that makes the following sentence grammatically correct.
Dr. Watson shook his head in bemusement at _____ explanation of his deductive reasoning skills.
    A. Sherlock Holmes'
    B. Sherlock Holme's
    C. Sherlock Holmes's
    D. Sherlock Holmes

16. Select the word or phrase that makes the following sentence grammatically correct.
The detective novel was so well written that Linus was completely shocked by the _____ solution.
    A. mysteries
    B. mystery's
    C. mysteries'
    D. mysterie's

17. Select the word or phrase that makes the following sentence grammatically correct.
Both Hugo and Camille _____ members of their local rotary club and frequently participate in the annual auction to raise money for charity.
    A. is
    B. was
    C. were
    D. are

18. Select the combination of words that makes the following sentence grammatically correct.
The coach tried to motivate his team by saying, "This year we will _____ to the challenge and _____ the bar for what we can accomplish together."
    A. rise, raise
    B. raise, raise
    C. raise, rise
    D. rise, rise

19. Select the combination of words that makes the following sentence grammatically correct.
Do not _____ down just yet; I need to _____ new sheets on that bed.
    A. lay, lay
    B. lay, lie
    C. lie, lie
    D. lie, lay

20. Select the combination of words that makes the following sentence grammatically correct.
_____ car has broken down, so _____ going to go to Evan's house and stay _____ until the car is repaired.
    A. their, they're, there
    B. they're, their, they're
    C. there, they're, their
    D. there, their, there

21. Select the combination of words that makes the following sentence grammatically correct.
_____ the two of us, I don't think there's much intelligence _____ all ten of the board members.
    A. among, among
    B. among, between
    C. between, among
    D. between, between

22. Select the punctuation that makes the following sentence grammatically correct.
    A. The committee will discuss the different options for the new park at the following meetings March 19th and March 26th.
    B. The committee will discuss the different options for the new park at the following meetings; March 19th and March 26th.
    C. The committee will discuss the different options for the new park at the following meetings: March 19th and March 26th.
    D. The committee will discuss the different options for the new park at the following meetings, March 19th and March 26th.

23. Select the punctuation that makes the following sentence grammatically correct.
    A. Margot's business travels have taken her to Topeka Kansas El Paso Texas and San Diego California.
    B. Margot's business travels have taken her to Topeka, Kansas, El Paso, Texas, and San Diego, California.
    C. Margot's business travels have taken her to Topeka Kansas, El Paso Texas, and San Diego California.
    D. Margot's business travels have taken her to Topeka, Kansas; El Paso, Texas; and San Diego, California.

24. Select the punctuation that makes the following sentence grammatically correct.
    A. Honestly Mateo what you're suggesting is impossible.
    B. Honestly, Mateo what you're suggesting is impossible.
    C. Honestly Mateo; what you're suggesting is impossible.
    D. Honestly, Mateo: what you're suggesting is impossible.

25. Select the combination of words that makes the following sentence grammatically correct.
_____ Marine, no one else wanted to go with Elsa and get some sun _____ the pool.
    A. beside, besides
    B. besides, beside
    C. beside, beside
    D. besides, besides

26. Select the punctuation that makes the following sentence grammatically correct.
    A. The more time we have to complete the project the better we will be.
    B. The more time we have to complete the project; the better we will be.
    C. The more time we have to complete the project: the better we will be.
    D. The more time we have to complete the project, the better we will be.

27. Select the punctuation that makes the following sentence grammatically correct.
    A. Jeannette, the guests will be arriving at what time
    B. Jeannette, the guests will be arriving at what time?
    C. Jeannette, the guests will be arriving at what time…
    D. Jeannette, the guests will be arriving at what time.

28. Select the word or phrase that makes the following sentence grammatically correct.
Either Eleanor or Patrick _____ given the job of picking up the ice for the party.
    A. should
    B. are
    C. was
    D. were

29. Select the word or phrase that makes the following sentence grammatically correct.
Edgar _____ to be there, but the trains were delayed by several hours.
    A. had liked
    B. would like
    C. was liking
    D. would have liked

30. Select the word or phrase that makes the following sentence grammatically correct.
If I _____ more diligent, I would tackle my housework in a more timely manner.
    A. were
    B. are
    C. am
    D. was

31. Select the word or phrase that makes the following sentence grammatically correct.
She insisted that the children _____ inside the house no later than four o'clock.
    A. will be
    B. be
    C. are
    D. were

32. Select the word or phrase that makes the following sentence grammatically correct.
The car needs _____ before we leave for our road trip.
    A. cleaned
    B. to clean
    C. cleaning
    D. to be cleaned

33. Select the word or phrase that makes the following sentence grammatically correct.
Knowing the impending danger, he went forward _____ and with great care.
    A. cautiously
    B. caution
    C. cautious
    D. cautioned

34. Select the word or phrase that makes the following sentence grammatically correct.
She assured the doctor that she felt _____ enough to take the vacation that she had been planning.
    A. good
    B. better
    C. well
    D. best

35. Select the word or phrase that makes the following sentence grammatically correct.
The town's one-hundred-year anniversary was a _____ event; even the state governor showed up to shake a few hands and congratulate the residents.
    A. important
    B. real important
    C. really important
    D. more important

36. Select the word or phrase that makes the following sentence grammatically correct.
Cedric was feeling weak because he _____ food all day.
    A. had any
    B. barely had any
    C. had barely no
    D. had barely any

37. Select the combination of words that makes the following sentence grammatically correct.
Meg was _____ than Beth and Jo, but Amy was considered to be the _____ of the four March girls.
    A. prettier, prettier
    B. prettier, prettiest
    C. prettiest, prettier
    D. prettiest, prettiest

38. Select the word or phrase that makes the following sentence grammatically correct.
For Thomas, seeing the live concert at the stadium was _____ and life-changing experience.
    A. the most unique
    B. a unique
    C. the uniquest
    D. a more unique

39. Select the combination of words that makes the following sentence grammatically correct.
He refused to consider _____ which route to the store would be best so he would not go _____ than necessary.
    A. farther, further
    B. farther, farther
    C. further, further
    D. further, farther

40. Select the combination of words that makes the following sentence grammatically correct.
Zenaida felt _____ that the child was doing so _____ in the math class.
    A. bad, bad
    B. badly, bad
    C. bad, badly
    D. badly, badly

41. Select the combination of words that makes the following sentence grammatically correct.
Jerome put the matter to the _____ for the consideration, assured that they would offer the _____ he so desperately needed.
    A. council, counsel
    B. council, council
    C. counsel, counsel
    D. counsel, council

42. Select the combination of words that makes the following sentence grammatically correct.
Please _____ me on the best choice for a contractor; I have so many options, and I am in need of sound _____.
    A. advise, advice
    B. advice, advise
    C. advice, advice
    D. advise, advise

43. Select the combination of words that makes the following sentence grammatically correct.
Our true emotions can often _____ us. That's what the poet was trying to _____ to in the romantic ballad.
    A. allude, allude
    B. elude, elude
    C. allude, elude
    D. elude, allude

44. Select the word or phrase that makes the following sentence grammatically correct.
Because Carl's truck broke down, he had to take four different _____ to get to work.
    A. busses
    B. buses
    C. bus
    D. bus's

45. Select the punctuation that makes the following sentence grammatically correct.
    A. The professor lectured on Pushkin: Today most scholars recognize that The Bronze Horseman both reveres Peter the Great and calls into question his tyrannical behavior.
    B. The professor lectured on Pushkin: "Today most scholars recognize that the poem The Bronze Horseman both reveres Peter the Great and calls into question his tyrannical behavior."
    C. The professor lectured on Pushkin: "Today most scholars recognize that the poem The Bronze Horseman both reveres Peter the Great and calls into question his tyrannical behavior."
    D. The professor lectured on Pushkin: "Today most scholars recognize that the poem "The Bronze Horseman" both reveres Peter the Great and calls into question his tyrannical behavior".

46. Which word is *not* spelled correctly in the context of the following sentence?
When they hurried the magnificent conveyance along, they were sure that they would be victoryous.
    A. hurried
    B. magnificent
    C. conveyance
    D. victoryous

47. Which word is *not* spelled correctly in the context of the following sentence?
Professor Rinkie told the story but preferred omitting the forgettable occurence with the horses.
    A. preferred
    B. omitting
    C. forgettable
    D. occurence

48. Choose the word or words that best fill the blank.
Marty did not realize until he arrived to perform in Philadelphia that he had left his guitar in Pittsburgh; _____, he was fortunate to find a music store that agreed to rent him one for the evening.
    A. however
    B. because
    C. after
    D. while

49. Choose the sentence that is correct and most clearly written.
    A. The novelist David Markson is known for his experimental works, such as "This Is Not a Novel."
    B. Experimental works such as "This Is Not a Novel" have been wrote by David Markson.
    C. Novelist David Markson is knew for his experimental works, such as "This Is Not a Novel."
    D. David Markson is a novelist who is known for experimentation his works include "This Is Not a Novel."

50. Choose the sentence that is correct and most clearly written.
    A. I intended to mow the yard, but I wanted to wait until evening when it are cooler.
    B. I intended to mow the yard, but I wanted to wait until evening when it would be cooler.
    C. I intended to mow the yard, but not until it getting cooler in the evening.
    D. I intended to mow the yard, but I waits until evening when it was cooler.

Section 4. Mathematics

Number of Questions: **50**
Time Limit: **50 Minutes**

1. 75% of 500
   A. 365
   B. 375
   C. 387
   D. 390

2. (7 x 5) + (8 x 2) =
   A. 51
   B. 57
   C. 85
   D. 560

3. (8 ÷ 2) (12 ÷ 3) =
   A. 1
   B. 8
   C. 12
   D. 16

4. Which number is a factor of 36?
   A. 5
   B. 7
   C. 8
   D. 9

5. 75 x 34 =
   A. 1200
   B. 2050
   C. 2550
   D. 3100

6. x + 372 = 853, x =
   A. 455
   B. 481
   C. 520
   D. 635

7. Convert .25 into fraction form.
   A. ¼
   B. ½
   C. 1/8
   D. 2/3

8. 0.85 =
    A. 13/15
    B. 17/20
    C. 18/19
    D. 19/22

9. Which fraction is closest to 2/3 without going over?
    A. 6/13
    B. 7/12
    C. 11/16
    D. 9/12

10. A circle graph is used to show the percent of patient types that a hospital sees. How many degrees of the circle should the graph show if 1/3 of the patient type is pediatric?
    A. 90 degrees
    B. 120 degrees
    C. 220 degrees
    D. 360 degrees

11. A traveler on vacation spent $ 25 at the grocery store the first week of school; the next two weeks he spent $ 52; and the last week he spent $34. What was his average food expenditure while he was on vacation?
    A. $ 37.00
    B. $ 38.25
    C. $ 40.75
    D. $ 52.00

12. 437.65 – 325.752 =
    A. 111.898
    B. 121.758
    C. 122.348
    D. 133.053

13. 43.3 x 23.03 =
    A. 997.199
    B. 999.999
    C. 1010.03
    D. 1111.01

14. After going on diet for two weeks, you have lost 6% of you weight. Your original weight was 157 lbs. What do you weigh now?
    A. 132 lbs
    B. 135.48 lbs
    C. 144.98 lbs
    D. 147.58 lbs

15. In order for a school to allow a vending machine to be placed next to the cafeteria, 65% of the school's population must ask for it. If 340 of the school's 650 students have requested the vending machines, how many more are needed to get the vending machines?
   A. 75
   B. 83
   C. 89
   D. 99

16. Round this number to the nearest hundredths 390.24657
   A. 400
   B. 390.247
   C. 390.25
   D. 390.2

17. To get 1 as an answer, you must multiply 4/5 by
   A. 5/4
   B. ½
   C. 1
   D. ¼

18. While working, patient's sodium intake was 300 mg on Monday, 1240 mg on Tuesday, 900 mg on Wednesday and Friday, and 1500 on Thursday. What was the average intake of sodium while the patient was at work?
   A. 476 mg
   B. 754 mg
   C. 968 mg
   D. 998 mg

19. Which of the following numbers is correctly rounded to the nearest tenth?
   A. 3.756 rounds to 3.76
   B. 4.567 rounds to 4.5
   C. 6.982 rounds to 7.0
   D. 54.32 rounds to 54.4

20. Which of the following fraction equal 0.625
   A. 3/4
   B. 5/6
   C. 5/8
   D. 2/3

21. A solution contains 6% calcium. How many milliliters of solution can be made from 50 ml of calcium?
   A. 833
   B. 952
   C. 1054
   D. 2000

22. 8.7 x 23.3 equals:
   A. 202.71
   B. 2027.1
   C. 212.71
   D. 2127.1

23. 134.5 Divided by 5 equals:
    A. 26.9
    B. 25.9
    C. 23.9
    D. 22.9

24. 23/3 =
    A. 6 2/3
    B. 7 1/3
    C. 7 2/3
    D. 8 1/3

25. 4500 + 3422 + 3909 =
    A. 12,831
    B. 12,731
    C. 11,831
    D. 11,731

26. 14,634 + 7,377
    A. 21,901
    B. 21,911
    C. 22,011
    D. 22,901

27. 9,645 - 6,132
    A. 2,513
    B. 2,517
    C. 3,412
    D. 3,513

28. 893 x 64
    A. 54,142
    B. 56,822
    C. 56,920
    D. 57,152

29. $97\overline{)29294}$

    A. 302
    B. 322
    C. 3002
    D. 3022

30. $\frac{38}{100}$ as a decimal
    A. 0.38
    B. 0.038
    C. 3.8
    D. 0.0038

31. 6.8 + 11.3+ 0.06
    A. 17.16
    B. 17.70
    C. 18.16
    D. 18.70

32. 0.28 x 0.17
    A. 0.2260
    B. 0.4760
    C. 0.0226
    D. 0.0476

33. Which numeral is in the thousandths place in 0.3874?
    A. 3
    B. 8
    C. 7
    D. 4

34. What is the equivalent decimal number for five hundred twelve thousandths?
    A. 0.512
    B. 0.0512
    C. 5120.
    D. 0.00512

35. $3\frac{1}{8} + 6 + \frac{3}{7} =$
    A. 9 31/56
    B. 9 1/2
    C. 9 21/56
    D. 9 7/8

36. $4\frac{1}{7} - 2\frac{1}{2} =$
    A. 2 5/14
    B. 1 5/14
    C. 1 9/14
    D. 2 9/14

37. $1\frac{1}{4} \times 3\frac{2}{5} \times 1\frac{2}{3} =$
    A. 7 1/12
    B. 5 5/6
    C. 6 7/12
    D. 8 11/15

38. $\frac{3}{5} \div \frac{1}{2} =$
    A. 1 1/5
    B. 3/10
    C. 1 7/10
    D. 4/5

39. Which of the following is correct?

A. $\frac{4}{7} = \frac{12}{21}$

B. $\frac{3}{4} = \frac{12}{20}$

C. $\frac{5}{8} = \frac{15}{32}$

D. $\frac{7}{9} = \frac{28}{35}$

40. Find N for the following:

$$\frac{n}{7} = \frac{18}{21}$$

A. 3

B. 4

C. 5

D. 6

41. Reduce $\frac{14}{98}$ to lowest terms.

A. $\frac{7}{49}$

B. $\frac{2}{14}$

C. $\frac{1}{7}$

D. $\frac{3}{8}$

42. Express $\frac{68}{7}$ as a mixed fraction.

A. $9\frac{5}{7}$

B. $8\frac{4}{7}$

C. $9\frac{3}{7}$

D. $8\frac{6}{7}$

43. Thirty six hundredths as a percent.

A. 36%

B. .36%

C. .036%

D. 3.6%

44. 3= (? %) of 60

A. 5

B. 9

C. 15

D. 20

45. 1 is what percent of 25?

A. 1%

B. 2%

C. 3%

D. 4%

46. Three eighths of forty equals:
    A. 15
    B. 20
    C. 22
    D. 24

47. $\frac{1}{3} = (?)\% \times \frac{5}{6}$
    A. 10
    B. 20
    C. 30
    D. 40

48. 3:15 as a percentage
    A. 5%
    B. .05%
    C. 2%
    D. 20%

49. $\frac{3}{12}$ as a percentage
    A. .25%
    B. .04%
    C. 25%
    D. 40%

50. 8% as a reduced common fraction
    A. $\frac{2}{50}$
    B. $\frac{4}{5}$
    C. $\frac{2}{5}$
    D. $\frac{2}{25}$

Section 5. Biology

| Number of Questions: **25** |
| Time Limit: **25 Minutes** |

1. Which chemicals are responsible for conveying an impulse along a nerve cell?
    A. Sodium and potassium
    B. Calcium
    C. Actin and myosin
    D. Phosphorus

2. What type of genetic mutation occurs when a piece of DNA breaks off the chromosome and attaches to a different chromosome?
    A. Nondisjunction
    B. Translocation
    C. Deletion
    D. Crossing over

3. What is the first line of defense against invading bacteria?
    A. The skin
    B. Macrophages
    C. T-cells
    D. Lymphocytes

4. What is the purpose of capping the 5' end of mRNA?
    A. To signal the end of the mRNA strand
    B. To prepare it to attach to the complementary DNA strand
    C. To protect the end of the strand from degradation
    D. There is no known reason for capping the end of an mRNA strand

5. During what process does hydrolysis occur to provide electrons to chlorophyll, which subsequently absorb energy?
    A. Light-dependent reactions of photosynthesis
    B. Light-independent reactions of photosynthesis
    C. Calvin cycle
    D. Krebs cycle

6. What is the process called when root hairs capture water and move it upwards into the rest of the plant?
    A. Photosynthesis
    B. Diffusion
    C. Active transport
    D. Transpiration

7. Which plant hormone causes fruit to ripen?
    A. Auxins
    B. Cytokinins
    C. Ethylene
    D. Abscisic Acid

8. What is thigmotropism?
    A. Growth of plant materials toward light
    B. Growth of leaves and stems opposite to the pull of gravity
    C. Growth toward a source of nutrition
    D. Growth of plant structures in response to contact with a physical structure

9. What is the purpose of the stigma?
    A. To gather pollen
    B. To attract pollinators like birds and bees
    C. To nourish the fertilized ovum
    D. To produce pollen

10. Organisms with the same _____ are most closely related.
    A. order
    B. genus
    C. family
    D. class

11. What are the first life forms to colonize a new area called?
    A. Primary producers
    B. Pioneer species
    C. Primary consumers
    D. Primary succession

12. Which of the following fibers is not found in the cytoskeleton?
    A. Microtubules
    B. Microfilaments
    C. Glycoproteins
    D. Intermediate filaments

13. Which biome is characterized by a population of cone-bearing trees?
    A. Tropical forest
    B. Tundra
    C. Temperate deciduous forest
    D. Coniferous forest

14. Which of the following is an example of an abiotic factor?
    A. Local vegetation
    B. Sunlight
    C. Endemic populations
    D. Ecosystem

15. Detritivores eat only what type of matter?
    A. Plants
    B. Animals
    C. Both plants and animals
    D. Dead and decaying matter

16. What type of population curve is produced once exponential growth is leveling off?
    A. S-curve
    B. J-curve
    C. K-curve
    D. R-curve

17. When one partner benefits and the other is harmed, what symbiotic relationship is formed?
    A. Mutualism
    B. Commensalism
    C. Parasitism
    D. Predation

18. In mice, brown fur is the dominant trait, and the recessive trait is white fur. In a cross between two heterozygous mice, how many offspring will be white if 24 mice result from the cross?
    A. 6
    B. 12
    C. 18
    D. 24

19. You are crossing fruit flies with two distinct traits: eye color and the presence/absence of wings. Having red eyes and the presence of wings are both dominant traits, while the recessive phenotypes are white eyes and the absence of wings. If you are crossing two flies that are heterozygous for both traits, what fraction of flies would you expect to have wings and white eyes?
    A. 0/16
    B. 1/16
    C. 3/16
    D. 9/16

20. Which of the following is true about sex-linked traits?
    A. They never occur in females
    B. They occur rarely in females
    C. The trait appears on the Y chromosome
    D. Sons usually inherit the trait from their father

21. Which of the following is not found on the exterior of most prokaryotic cells?
    A. Pili
    B. Flagella
    C. Capsule
    D. Plasma membrane

22. Which of the following will affect enzymatic activity?
    A. Temperature
    B. Amount of water
    C. Form of the enzyme
    D. Concentration of fatty acids

23. Transcription of the genetic material occurs when:
    A. DNA is copied identically to be distributed to its daughter cells
    B. DNA is copied into the complementary form of mRNA
    C. DNA is converted to the coded protein
    D. the message is edited into a form that the ribosome can understand

24. Where does translation occur?
    A. In the nucleus
    B. In the centrosome
    C. In the ribosome
    D. In the cytoplasm

25. What type of selection is occurring when the intermediate trait, not either of the extremes, is the driving force?
    A. Divergent Evolution
    B. Disruptive Evolution
    C. Directional Selection
    D. Stabilizing Selection

Section 6. Chemistry

| Number of Questions: **25** |
| Time Limit: **25 Minutes** |

1. The concentration of hydrogen ions in a neutral solution is:
   A. 7
   B. 10^7
   C. 10^{-7}
   D. 10^{-14}

2. What will adding an acid to a base will yield?
   A. A neutral solution
   B. A salt
   C. An acid
   D. A base

3. Alcohols have which common structure?
   A. A benzene ring
   B. A carbon atom with a double bond to an oxygen atom and a single bond to a hydroxyl group
   C. A nitrogen bond which is also bonded to other carbon atoms
   D. A hydroxyl group

4. Which of the following is an example of a primary amine?

   A.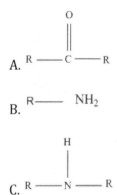

   B.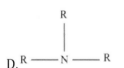

   C.

   D.

5. Which of the following is not true of hydrocarbons?
   A. They are volatile
   B. They have low boiling points
   C. Nonpolar/London dispersion forces hold the hydrocarbon together
   D. Most hydrocarbons are solids

6. What is the primary difference between ketones and aldehydes?
    A. Ketones contain two functional groups and a double-bonded oxygen attached to a central carbon atom, while aldehydes contain only one functional group, a hydrogen atom, and a double-bonded oxygen atom bonded to the central carbon.
    B. Aldehydes contain two functional groups and a double-bonded oxygen attached to a central carbon atom, while ketones contain only one functional group, a hydrogen atom, and a double-bonded oxygen atom bonded to the central carbon.
    C. Ketones are polar substances, and aldehydes are nonpolar substances.
    D. Aldehydes are polar substances, and ketones are nonpolar substances.

7. What type of organic reaction occurs when water is released as two functional groups bond together?
    A. Substitution
    B. Hydrolysis
    C. Condensation
    D. Radical reaction

8. Which of the following is the Lewis Dot structure for NO_3^-?

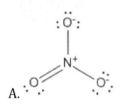
A.

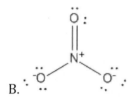
B.

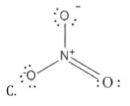
C.

    D. All of the above

9. What is the release of a massive amount of energy caused by the bombarding and splitting of a nucleus by a neutron called?
    A. Positron emission
    B. Nuclear fission
    C. Controlled fusion
    D. Electron capture

10. How many valence electrons do the noble gases contain in their valence shell?
    A. 2
    B. 4
    C. 6
    D. 8

11. What is one mole equal to?
    A. 6.02×10^{23} units
    B. 6.02×10^{-23} units
    C. 6.02×10^{10} units
    D. 6.02×10^{-10} units

12. A patient has a temperature of 99.1 degrees Fahrenheit. What is the temperature in Kelvin?
    A. 372 Kelvin
    B. 310 Kelvin
    C. 273 Kelvin
    D. 37.3 Kelvin

13. A sample of O_2 gas is heated from 35°C to 100°C. The final pressure of the gas is 2.5 atm. What was the initial pressure of the gas if the volume of the container remained constant through the heating process?
    A. 0.875 atm
    B. 1 atm
    C. 7.1 atm
    D. 10 atm

14. Increasing the volume of a gas will:
    A. decrease the temperature.
    B. increase the number of moles of the gas.
    C. decrease the pressure of the gas.
    D. make the gas more volatile.

15. A covalent bond occurs when:
    A. two atoms bond together
    B. one electron transfers from one atom to another, forming two ions
    C. both bonding electrons come from the same atom
    D. an electron pair is shared between two atoms, creating the bond

16. Which of the following is released during a combustion reaction?
    A. Water
    B. Heat
    C. Oxygen
    D. Electrons

17. Which of the following is an example of a colligative property?
    A. Boiling point depression
    B. Freezing point elevation
    C. Freezing point depression
    D. Elevation of vapor pressure

18. After balancing the following reaction, what is the coefficient of the molecule of water?
$C_6H_{12}O_6 + O_2 \rightarrow CO_2 + H_2O$
    A. 1
    B. 2
    C. 3
    D. 6

19. According to the second law of thermodynamics:
    A. energy is neither created nor destroyed
    B. entropy is always increasing in the universe
    C. the entropy of a crystal at absolute zero temperature is zero
    D. enthalpy increases within a universe

20. When two atoms are triple bonded to each other, how many electrons do they share?
    A. 1
    B. 2
    C. 3
    D. 6

21. Hydrophobic molecules are:
    A. nonpolar
    B. polar
    C. dipolar
    D. unipolar

22. Which of the following is NOT an example of a monosaccharide?
    A. Glucose
    B. Fructose
    C. Sucrose
    D. Mannose

23. An exergonic reaction is one that:
    A. absorbs energy
    B. releases energy
    C. involves the addition of water
    D. involves the transfer of electrons occurs between reactants

24. What is the difference between an Arrhenius base and a Brønsted-Lowery base?
    A. An Arrhenius base accepts protons, and the Brønsted-Lowery base donates hydrogen ions
    B. The Arrhenius base releases hydroxide molecules, while the Brønsted-Lowery base donates hydrogen ions
    C. The Arrhenius base releases hydroxide ions, and the Brønsted-Lowery base accepts hydrogen ions
    D. The Arrhenius base accepts hydrogen ions, and the Brønsted-Lowery base releases hydroxide molecules

25. What are the weak forces that exist between all molecules called?
    A. London dispersion forces
    B. Dipole-dipole forces
    C. Hydrogen forces
    D. Chemical bonds

Section 7. Anatomy and Physiology	Number of Questions: 25
	Time Limit: **25 Minutes**

1. Which structure in the brain is responsible for arousal and maintenance of consciousness?
    A. The midbrain
    B. The reticular activating system
    C. The diencephalon
    D. The limbic system

2. The triceps reflex:
    A. forces contraction of the triceps and extension of the arm
    B. forces contraction of the biceps, relaxation of the biceps, and arm extension
    C. causes the triceps to contract, causing the forearm to supinate and flex
    D. causes the triceps to relax and the upper arm to pronate and extend

3. Which cranial nerve is responsible for hearing and balance?
    A. CN III
    B. CN V
    C. CN VIII
    D. CN XII

4. Which gland is responsible for the regulation of calcium levels?
    A. The parathyroid glands
    B. The pituitary gland
    C. The adrenal glands
    D. The pancreas

5. Which hormone is predominantly produced during the luteal phase of the menstrual cycle?
    A. Estrogen
    B. Luteinizing hormone
    C. Follicle stimulating hormone
    D. Progesterone

6. The pancreas secretes what hormone in response to low blood glucose levels?
    A. Insulin
    B. Glucagon
    C. Somatostatin
    D. Amylase

7. Which layer of the heart contains striated muscle fibers for contraction of the heart?
    A. Pericardium
    B. Epicardium
    C. Endocardium
    D. Myocardium

8. Which part of the cardiac conduction system is the most distal from the initial impulse generation and actually conducts the charge throughout the heart tissue?
   A. SA node
   B. AV node
   C. Perkinje fibers
   D. Bundle of His

9. Which blood vessel carries oxygenated blood back to the heart?
   A. Pulmonary vein
   B. Pulmonary artery
   C. Aorta
   D. Superior vena cava

10. Which granulocyte is most likely to be elevated during an allergic response?
    A. Neutrophil
    B. Monocyte
    C. Eosinophil
    D. Basophil

11. Which vitamin is essential for proper formation of clotting factors?
    A. Vitamin A
    B. Vitamin K
    C. Vitamin B
    D. Vitamin C

12. Afferent lymph vessels carry lymph:
    A. toward the spleen
    B. away from the spleen
    C. toward the lymph node
    D. away from the lymph node

13. Cricoid cartilage is found on the:
    A. alveoli
    B. bronchioles
    C. bronchi
    D. trachea

14. Which of the following is not found in the mediastinum?
    A. Xiphoid process
    B. Thymus
    C. Trachea
    D. Vagus nerve

15. What is the proper order of the divisions of the small intestine as food passes through the gastrointestinal tract?
    A. Ileum, duodenum, jejunum
    B. Duodenum, Ileum, jejunum
    C. Duodenum, jejunum, ileum
    D. Ileum, jejunum, duodenum

16. The primary function of gastrin is to:
    A. inhibit gastric secretion of other hormones
    B. stimulate secretion of pancreatic enzymes
    C. break down lipids
    D. stimulate secretion of gastric enzymes and motility of the stomach

17. The majority of nutrient absorption occurs in the:
    A. mouth
    B. stomach
    C. small intestine
    D. large intestine

18. What is the approximate average bladder capacity in an adult?
    A. 500 ml
    B. 1000 ml
    C. 1500 ml
    D. 2000 ml

19. Which hormone regulates the amount of urine output?
    A. Angiotension I
    B. Angiotension II
    C. Anti-diuretic hormone
    D. Renin

20. Where is the interstitial fluid found?
    A. In the blood and lymphatic vessels
    B. In the tissues around cells
    C. In the cells
    D. In the ventricles of the brain

21. Which range represents the normal pH of the body fluids ?
    A. 7.05 to 7.15
    B. 7.15 to 7.25
    C. 7.25 to 7.35
    D. 7.35 to 7.45

22. What lab values would you expect to see in a patient with respiratory acidosis?
    A. Increased $PaCO_2$ and decreased pH
    B. Decreased $PaCO_2$ and decreased pH
    C. Increased HCO_3^- and decreased pH
    D. Decreased HCO_3^- and decreased pH

23. Which testicular cells secrete testosterone?
    A. Sertoli cells
    B. Leydig's cells
    C. Skene's glands
    D. Cowper's glands

24. Where does fertilization of an egg by a sperm cell occur?
    A. The ovary
    B. The uterus
    C. The cervix
    D. The fallopian tubes

25. Which cells are found in the skin and assist in boosting immune function?
    A. Melanocytes
    B. Reticular fibers
    C. Eccrine glands
    D. Langerhans cells

AnswerExplanations

ReadingComprehensionAnswerKeyandExplanations

1. B: The author's primary purpose is to inform the reader about the apparent increase in cases of rickets in developed nations. There is nothing about the essay that suggests persuasion, as the author is simply providing information rather than attempting to persuade the reader to agree with a certain position or opinion. The author provides information but does not necessarily analyze it too closely, so the author's purpose is not to analyze. Additionally, there is little in the essay that indicates a desire to entertain.

2. B: Based on the information at the end of the first paragraph and at the beginning of the second paragraph, the author's main point is that rickets has once again become a problem in some developed nations. (The author starts by noting that this disease is typically seen in nations where children face malnourishment, but that this has not occurred in developed nations for many decades.) Answer choice A suggests a persuasive argument that is not present within the essay. The author does make a final note at the end about rickets becoming a disease of the past, but this is more of a hopeful comment than a call to action. Answer choice C offers information that the author includes as part of the explanation about rickets, but it is supporting information and not the main point. The author singles out the United States and Great Britain but also refers to "other places" where the disease has surprised doctors with its reappearance. This suggests other countries besides the United States and Great Britain, so answer choice D cannot be correct.

3. C: The author clearly mentions the information that is in answer choices A, B, and D. The possibility of a phosphorus deficiency contributing to rickets is noted in the first paragraph. The fact that sunscreen has been identified as a possible vitamin D blocker is mentioned in the third paragraph. The fact that rickets has not been a problem in the United States since the Great Depression is also included in the first paragraph. The author says that *children* in Great Britain are identified as having low vitamin D levels, but there is no mention of vitamin D levels in adults in Great Britain. (This information is actually true, but it is not included in the essay, so answer choice C is correct.)

4. A: If rickets—at least in the United States—was usually a problem that accompanied poor nutrition, and rickets has not been a problem since the Great Depression, the reader can infer that the diet in the United States has improved since the Great Depression. There is nothing in the passage to suggest that people are already taking calcium and vitamin D supplements; in fact, the author notes that doctors are recommending it because people do not have enough calcium and vitamin D. (If they do not have enough, they cannot already be taking the supplements.) The author mentions that sunshine in Great Britain is often in short supply, but there is no discussion of sunshine in the United States. What is more, the author mentions Georgia and North Carolina, neither of which is known for being excessively overcast. And there is no discussion about children's play patterns in the United States, so it cannot be inferred that children in the United States have a vitamin D deficiency because they spend too much time indoors and/or wear too much sunscreen. This discussion is limited to the third paragraph, about Great Britain.

5. D: The author states the exact opposite of the information in answer choice D: far from discouraging breastfeeding, doctors still recommend it. They just encourage nursing mothers to have their vitamin D levels checked and to add a supplement if the levels are low. The author contrasts the developed nations with those that traditionally have poor nutrition and where children suffer from rickets. Developing nations tend to fall into the category of the "third world," so answer choice A is a safe inference. The author includes the information from answer choice B in the final paragraph, so this cannot be correct. Similarly, the author notes in the first sentence of the final paragraph that rickets is not yet considered an epidemic in developed nations but that doctors are concerned about seeing it at all.

6. A: Given the shift in focus from the second paragraph to the third, it is safe to assume that the cause of rickets in Great Britain is linked more to low vitamin D than to low calcium. In fact, the author states outright that doctors in Great Britain believe the cases of rickets are "connected largely to low vitamin D levels." That sunscreen is connected to blocking vitamin D is mentioned, but nothing is said about whether doctors recommend that children wear (or stop wearing) sunscreen. There is no discussion about nursing mothers in Great Britain, so it is impossible to infer anything about the levels of vitamin D in their breast milk. In the first paragraph, low levels of phosphorus are noted as a possible cause of rickets; it is also mentioned that "some researchers" believe this. The word *some* is too vague to determine in any quantity, so it is impossible to say with any certainty if "most researchers" disagree with this.

7. D: In the first paragraph, the author clearly connects rickets with poor nutrition. The author also mentions a time (the Great Depression) when there was poor nutrition in the United States. This would suggest that the term *developed nations* refers to those nations where the citizens have access to adequate nutritional options. There is no mention of a "status quo" anywhere in the passage, so answer choice A makes no sense. Additionally, there is no discussion of politics and economics, so answer choice B cannot be correct. As Great Britain is included among the developed nations but is also noted for having limited sunshine, answer choice C is also incorrect.

8. A: Among the available answer choices, only the word *abundant* makes real sense in the context of the paragraph: Great Britain is not known for having abundant amounts of sunshine. The word *small* makes no sense in the paragraph, since the author is claiming that there is often limited sunshine. The word *expected* does not work, since there is no mention about the amount of sunshine that would be expected. The word *appropriate* does not work, since it is difficult to say whether a certain amount of sunshine is appropriate.

9. A: In the final paragraph, the author simply provides information for preventing and eliminating rickets. Again, this is not a persuasive essay, but the final paragraph is not persuasive in tone. It is largely informative, and the essay would feel incomplete without it. After all, if the essay ended after the third paragraph, the reader would likely wonder about the solution to the problem of rickets. The author says nothing about developing nations in the final paragraph; in fact, the focus is largely on ridding developed nations of a disease that has returned. The author mentions nursing mothers in the final paragraph, but this is in conjunction with the other possible solutions; so the final paragraph is clearly not focused only on nursing mothers. And answer choice D is too broad for the information in the final paragraph. The author suggests possible options for getting rid of rickets in developed nations, but there is little to infer a "world without rickets" from the information in the paragraph.

10. C: The author focuses on three primary recommendations in the final paragraph: children getting a little sunshine each day (to ensure some vitamin D absorption), people taking vitamin D and calcium supplements, and nursing mothers having their vitamin D levels checked. Limiting television and video games among children is not included as a recommendation, so answer choice C is correct.

11. C: The last sentence of the first paragraph shapes the main idea of the essay: doctors and researchers are concerned about the long-term problems that might result from the chicken pox vaccine. Additionally, the final sentence in the essay notes that there is "ongoing debate about the value of the chicken pox vaccine." These statements offer a clear sense of focus for the essay. The passage does not say that getting the chicken pox vaccine can cause problems with shingles later in life, but this is a supporting point in the passage and not the main idea. Similarly, the author mentions that an increasing number of people in the United States are getting the chicken pox vaccine, but this is a fact the author uses to shape the main point and not the main point itself. The author notes that many children contract chicken pox, but the only mention of adults is in connection with shingles. In fact, there are adults that catch chicken pox, but this is not mentioned in the essay, nor can it be identified as the main point.

12. D: The author's primary purpose is simply to inform the reader about the concerns that many doctors and researchers have about the chicken pox vaccine. The author does not take a clear stand on the issue, and the author does not attempt to persuade the reader either way. The author includes information that analyzes the problem, but the overall focus is on providing information rather than on analyzing. And while the tone of the essay is occasionally playful, the topic is not, so it cannot be said that the author's purpose is to entertain—particularly on so serious a subject.

13. A: The author refers to epidemiologists in conjunction with the potential outbreak of shingles among the people in the United States. This would suggest that an epidemiologist studies diseases among a population. (Looking more closely at the word, the reader can also see a connection to the word *epidemic*, which is the outbreak of disease among a large number of people in a population.) There is no mention of internal organs anywhere in the essay, and as anyone who has had chicken pox knows it reveals itself at the topical level; answer choice B cannot be correct. Chicken pox is indeed a virus (*varicella*), and it is most common among children, but the word *epidemiologist* is not used anywhere near the specific discussion of children and viruses, so answer choice C is too great a stretch. Similarly, the author mentions the outbreak of shingles, but the word *problems* is itself a problem in answer choice D. Shingles is a *disease* that results from a *virus*. What is more, the author makes it clear that shingles is serious enough to go beyond a mere "adult problem," so answer choice D does not have enough support in the passage.

14. A: Nowhere in the passage does the author mention deaths in the United States as a result of chicken pox. The author does, however, note that shingles develops from the same virus as chicken pox. The author states quite clearly that some researchers and doctors believe *not* getting chicken pox might cause problems later on. And the author points out that shingles is a far more serious disease than chicken pox, in part because it attacks elderly adults whose health is already frail.

15. B: The author makes the connection between chicken pox and avoiding shingles: people who contract chicken pox in childhood develop a built-in immunity to shingles later in life. While chicken pox is inconvenient and it might be better to get it over with during childhood, the author says nothing to suggest this as a reason in favor of contracting chicken pox. Answer choice C gets part of the way there, but it does not offer the real reason for contracting chicken pox during childhood: the dormant virus helps *avoid contacting shingles*. And answer choice D is fairly absurd; one should not be in favor of contracting a disease just for the purpose of demonstrating the body's ability to develop a natural immunity to something else.

16. C: The author notes that contracting chicken pox means the individual always has the virus in his or her body. Being around others who have or have had chicken pox creates a kind of booster shot against the disease—just without the actual vaccine. It is a natural immunity boost against the virus, even as it remains in the body. Answer choice A presents a fairly backward way of looking at the issue. What is more, it does not identify the real reason for *being around others who have or have had the disease*, as explained in the correct answer choice, C. Answer choice B provides the desired side effect of catching chicken pox but does not answer the question that is posed. And answer choice D is the preferred result, but again it does not answer the specific question.

17. D: While the author explains that doctors and researchers are concerned about the long-term effects of the vaccine and continue to debate it, there is nothing in the passage to suggest that anyone is advising against it. The author says quite clearly that chicken pox is usually seen as a childhood disease, so it can be inferred that most people contract it during childhood. The author mentions that shingles affects adults over 60, and many of them already have weakened health. This would suggest that their age and state of health increases the problems that shingles brings with it. Finally, the author points out in the first paragraph that vaccines have been invaluable for ridding society of many serious diseases.

18. D: Question 18 requires a little analytical thinking. Avoiding the shingles has two primary parts to it: contracting chicken pox (preferably in childhood) and then being around those who have or have had chicken pox. Extensive vaccinations might not prevent some from catching chicken pox (primarily if they were not vaccinated), but this might mean that people are not around enough people who have had the disease to boost the immunity to it. Answer choice D, therefore, is correct. The author states that the amount of disease in the vaccine is not enough for those who have had chicken pox to boost their immunity to it (among those who have had the vaccine). The author does not, however, mention that the amount in the vaccine is not enough to prevent the shingles later on. Answer choice A cannot be correct. Answer choice B makes little sense. The fears of researchers should not be based on whether there are enough people to use for the study of a disease. Answer choice C has little connection to the question that is posed, so it too cannot be correct.

19. B: The author notes that epidemiologists project the possibility for over 20 million cases of shingles and about 5,000 deaths from the disease. Nothing is mentioned, however, about the time period over which this could occur. One year? Five years? Ten years? Without this information, it is difficult to know how serious of a problem this really is. (In reality, these numbers are projected over the course of fifty years, something that would greatly aid the reader in appreciating the information better.) The names of the researchers would make no difference to the reader's appreciation of the information. The detail about the countries where the vaccine is currently in use has little value for the reader, since these cases/deaths are projected in the United States. The information about the number of people currently vaccinated against chicken pox might be useful elsewhere in the essay, but it does very little to make the author's point stronger in the sentence that is mentioned.

20. C: As noted before, the author does not take a stand but rather focuses on providing information. As a result, the only valid inference from the final statement—when taken in the context of the entire essay—is that the ongoing debate means that researchers continue to evaluate and consider the long-term effects of the chicken pox vaccine. Nothing is said about researchers who advise against the vaccine; the only mention is that there is concern and debate. The final sentence notes only "ongoing debate," so there is not enough here (or in the rest of the essay) to infer that researchers believe the vaccine to cause more harm than good. The author says nothing about the number of people who have received or plan to receive the vaccine, so the reader cannot infer that the number of chicken pox vaccinations has decreased.

21. C: An expository composition *exposes* a subject matter by looking at it more closely and analyzing its significance. Additionally, the reader can determine the author's purpose through a process of elimination. As the author takes no clear stand on the issue and does not attempt to convince the reader to assume one side or the other, the passage cannot be persuasive. An investigative piece would require the subject matter to be a mystery that needs to be solved or a problem that needs to be revealed to the public. The author explores the topic and analyzes it more closely, but there is no major reveal within the passage. Finally, an advisory passage would be similar to a persuasive passage in that the author would encourage the reader to take a stand on the issue. As the author does not do that, the only possible answer choice is C.

22. D: The final two sentences of the passage present its main point. The World Health Organization agrees that the remaining samples of the smallpox vaccine should be destroyed, but those within the organization cannot agree about whether all of the samples should be destroyed and when the destruction should occur. Answer choice A cannot be correct because it suggests a persuasive tone that is not within the passage; the author presents information but does not take a stand on the issue. In the same way, answer choice B is incorrect; it offers the polar opposite view that is in answer choice A, but it is still persuasive in tone. And while the author suggests that the United States and Russia cannot agree about whether to destroy the samples, this small part of the passage cannot represent the main point.

23. B: This is something of a trick question that requires careful reading. The author notes that samples of the smallpox virus are still kept in laboratories in Russia. The author also points out that the Soviet Union collapsed in 1991, so it no longer exists. This means that the samples cannot be maintained in a nonexistent political entity. In all reality, the samples are likely to be in the same place in Russia that they were in the Soviet Union (i.e., in the same laboratory). But it is essential to note the relevance of detail in reading comprehension questions, and answer choice B offers a detail that cannot be described as part of the passage.

24. A: The word *consigned* has a range of meanings, depending on the context. It can mean everything from *transferred* to *assign*. In this context, it indicates that the virus has been *sent* to the dustbin of history. What is more, the other answer choices make little sense in the passage. It is illogical to say that the virus has been *refused* to the dustbin of history. Similarly, it cannot be said that the disease is *hidden* in/to the dustbin of history. The sentence indicates that the WHO instituted an inoculation program with the goal of getting rid of the disease among the general population, so it does not make any sense to say that they would want to *keep* it, at least outside of carefully guarded laboratories.

25. A: The last sentence of the second paragraph forges the link between the WHO's ongoing maintenance of the virus samples and the future: the samples provide the means of developing treatment and a vaccine in case of a bioterrorist attack. It makes little sense to argue that the WHO would retain the samples of the virus to prevent the actual attacks of bioterrorism; the relevance seems to be in the need for a response to bioterrorism. While the WHO might very well be interested in continuing research on the virus, there is little in the passage to indicate that this is the reason for retaining the samples. In fact, the author makes a much clearer link between maintaining the samples and responding to bioterrorism. And there is nothing in the passage to suggest that the WHO is prepared to institute a new vaccination program.

26. D: Far from arguing that the WHO is "confident" about the secret samples of the virus, the author makes the parenthetical remark that any unofficial samples were "never confirmed to be real." This does not mean, of course, that they do not exist, but it does suggest that the WHO is not necessarily confident about them. What is more, the author does not focus much on this issue, as the parenthetical remark would indicate. And all other answer choices reflect logical inferences from the passage. The author notes that 70 percent of those who contract smallpox survive; this means that the *majority* of people survive the virus. The author notes at the end of the passage that the WHO cannot agree about whether to destroy all of the remaining samples of the virus. And the author mentions at the beginning of the final paragraph that smallpox is one of the diseases that the WHO believes could be used for acts of bioterrorism.

27. C: In the last paragraph, the author mentions that some researchers—those who support the destruction of the samples—believe that it is no longer necessary to maintain them. This is because a vaccine is already in place to prevent outbreaks of smallpox. Answer choice A does not make much sense because the problem is the potential for outbreaks as a result of bioterrorism. Bioterrorism results not from natural causes of a disease but from deliberate acts of aggression. The disease might be obsolete in the sense of natural outbreaks, but it is not obsolete with regard to the possibility of bioterrorism. Answer choice B cannot be correct because the author makes no connection between the collapse of the Soviet Union in 1991 and the reduced risk of bioterrorism. In fact, the relevance of the researchers' concern suggests that bioterrorism remains a very real threat. Answer choice D goes against the author's statement in the last paragraph that most people are now susceptible to the virus; if they are susceptible, it would stand to reason that few people have been vaccinated.

28. B: Reading between the lines, it is possible to infer two things: there are very few people today who are vaccinated, and among those who were vaccinated during the WHO's inoculation program the effects of the vaccine have worn off. The author notes that the severity of smallpox can create side effects even for those who get the vaccine, but there is no mention about whether people are choosing to be (or not to be) vaccinated. As a result, answer choices A and C cannot be correct. Additionally, the author says little about the public response to smallpox, focusing instead on the concerns of the WHO and other researchers, so answer choice D cannot be correct.

29. D: Even without knowing the meaning of the phrase *at loggerheads*, the reader can deduce from the context that it indicates some kind of clash between the United States and Russia. The sentence states that, "Even the two nations that hold these final samples are at loggerheads about the issue." What is more, this follows the sentences that describe disagreement among scientists about whether to destroy the samples of smallpox virus. As a result, the reader can infer that the expression indicates a dispute of some kind. While the two nations might very well be considering their options, this expression does not offer the sense of disagreement that is implied within the passage. Similarly, the nations might be quietly discussing the issue and might be eager to arrive at a decision, but answer choices B and C do not provide the hint of dispute that is implied in this sentence, as well as the previous sentences.

30. B: The author makes the parenthetical remark that animals do not contract smallpox. At no point in the passage does the author reverse this statement or suggest that animals can contract smallpox, so answer choice B reflects a detail that is not a part of the passage. Answer choice A is incorrect because the author notes that the WHO was instrumental, and successful, in developing a vaccination program to combat smallpox; it also stands to reason that if the program was successful it must have been widespread, affecting many nations around the world. Answer choice B is incorrect because the author mentions in the first paragraph that loss of vision is a potential side effect of smallpox among those who survive. Answer choice D is incorrect because the author states that there were fears of unofficial samples in the hands not just of the Soviet government but of other governments as well.

31. D: The passage starts by providing information on the Black Death and then goes on to discuss the various theories about the cause of the disease. The tone is largely *explanatory*, in that the author explains the information to the reader. A process of elimination can also be useful in this case. There is little about the passage that suggests a *playful* tone. The author does not appear to be overly *concerned* at any point. And the word *definitive* indicates that something is the decisive or ultimate version. The author's tone cannot be described this way, as the author simply informs and explains but does not claim to know everything about the topic.

32. A: There are two parts to the passage, and the main idea should encompass these two parts: the Black Death was devastating for medieval people, and the exact cause or causes of the disease are still under debate. Answer choice B indicates a supporting detail within the second paragraph, but this alone is not enough to present the main point. Answer choice C offers information that is a small detail in the first paragraph; at the same time, answer choice C also goes beyond the information in the passage to suggest a call to action that is not a part of the author's purpose. And like answer choice B, answer choice D only gets half of the information right; it includes details from the first paragraph in the passage but omits the details in the second paragraph.

33. C: At no point does the author mention the Black Death outside of Europe. In fact, the information in answer choice C is correct (or partially correct, since the Black Death was believed to have spread *to* Europe as a result of trading vessels arriving *from* Asia). But it is not a part of the passage. The author does mention, however, that the Black Death reappeared in Europe at various times until the nineteenth century. The author indicates clearly that there remains debate about the cause of the Black Death. And the author states in the first paragraph that medieval doctors did not know what caused the Black Death and thus had no cure for it.

34. B: The author mentions that one theory about the cause of the Black Death notes that there is a similarity between the *spread* of the disease and the Ebola virus. This alone is not enough to suggest that the diseases are related; in fact, the author points out that this is a theory, disputed among scientists and historians, so the fact of a connection between the diseases cannot be inferred. In the last paragraph, the author mentions that the cause(s) of the Black Death remain uncertain. This suggests that there might very well be more than one cause of the disease, and answer choice A can be inferred. In the first paragraph, the author says that between 90 and 95 percent of those who contracted the disease died. This indicates that 5 to 10 percent of those infected survived, so answer choice C can be inferred. In the final sentence of the second paragraph, the author states that the Black Death "permanently changed Europe." Permanent changes have far-reaching effects, so answer choice D can be inferred.

35. A: The author indicates that there are two objections raised to the traditional theory of the bubonic plague: the appearance of the symptoms and the climate of Europe. The explanation about lower lymph nodes is part of the first objection, but this is not the only problem that some have with the flea-and-rat theory. The author mentions that anthrax from cattle has been raised as another alternative theory to the bubonic plague, but the author says nothing about current research seeing a relationship between the diseases. (Again, this is simply one theory among several.) The problem with fleas living long enough to infect so many victims is embedded in the mention of climate, but it too is not the only part of the objection and is thus not enough for a correct answer.

36. C: Question 36 asks the student to identify the author's use of punctuation and what it indicates. Parentheses can solve multiple purposes; in this case, they simply cordon off sentences that are an interesting side note within the discussion but do not fit perfectly into the author's primary flow of thought. The sentences follow from the discussion just before—about how medieval doctors were unsure of the cause—but they create a divergence without the parentheses. Using the parentheses allows the author to include this information while indicating to the reader that it is simply a quick side note. Parentheses seldom create emphasis. In fact, they are used more to minimize the impact of information than to highlight it. And because parentheses do not typically create emphasis, there is no reason to think that the author includes them to strengthen the main point. These brief historical details are more anecdotal than essential, and they do not represent important historical detail. Finally, there is no source noted within the parentheses, so there is no reason to believe that the author is including information from another source here.

37. B: In the first paragraph, the author states that the Black Death "struck and spread quickly," and in the second paragraph, the author points out that some have noticed a similarity between the *spread* of the Ebola virus and the *spread* of the Black Death. This would suggest that the former spreads quickly, just like the latter. While the author points out in the second paragraph that the cause or causes of the Black Death *might* never be known, there is nothing to suggest that it is *impossible* to know the cause or causes. The author says in the first paragraph that there has not been an outbreak of the Black Death since the nineteenth century. This is not enough, however, to assume that modern medicine has ensured another outbreak *will not* occur. The author writes in the first paragraph that medieval people killed cats, believing they were responsible for the Black Death. This suggests a superstitious approach to dealing with the disease. At the same time, the author makes no mention of medieval *doctors* killing cats and does not indicate that the doctors used superstitious approaches to treatment.

38. B: The author's purpose is twofold: to *inform* the reader about the problems that arise with swimmer's ear and to *advise* the reader about how to avoid it. At no point does the author *define* anything, and if there is nothing defined the author cannot *expand* on it. While the author clearly *presents* information, the passage is not *persuasive* in tone; after all, there is nothing to suggest that the author is trying to persuade the reader to believe or do something. Also, while the author does *explain* the details about swimmer's ear, there is little in the passage to indicate that the author is trying to *approve* anything.

39. D: The author says that people who get water in their ear while swimming run the risk of developing swimmer's ear. This is not a guarantee, however. Many people get water in their ear and never develop the condition. Answer choice D cannot be inferred. At the same time, the author says clearly that swimmer's ear results from the bacteria that is in the water making its way into the ear canal. The author notes in the first paragraph that swimmer's ear causes "a bit of swelling" and in the second paragraph that the condition results in the ear canal becoming "inflamed." Taken together, these indicate that swimmer's ear leads to a swelling of the ear canal. Additionally, in the first paragraph, the author notes that the condition is usually seen more as inconvenient than serious, and the author points out in the second paragraph that the problems associated with swimmer's ear can escalate and create more serious side effects.

40. A: Answer choice A is essentially true, but it is not a detail from the passage. Within the passage, the author links swimmer's ear and swimming pools but says nothing about other bodies of water. While the condition might be inferred (however vaguely) to come from other bodies of water, this fact is an implication and not a detail in any of the three paragraphs. The author states in the second paragraph that "otitis externa" is the official name for swimmer's ear. The author notes in the first paragraph that more than two million people in the United States suffer from swimmer's ear annually (and "more than two million" is definitely "over one million"). The author says in the second paragraph that swimmer's ear results from the bacteria in swimming water getting into the ear canal.

41. C: Question 41 asks only for an answer that is *based on the information in the passage*. In all reality, any of the answer choices might technically be true, but the only fact mentioned by the author is that the chlorine in swimming pools is not enough to keep up with all of the bacteria that develops from extra bodies in the water.

42. C: The author says clearly in the third paragraph that the "head-banging" routine (or shaking the head vigorously to release any water in the ear canal) is not advised and offers three options: alcohol to draw the water out, a towel to absorb the water in the ear canal, and a blow dryer.

43. A: Answer choice A is the most complete summary of the information in the passage, which is in two parts: the mysterious sweating sickness broke out in England in the fifteenth and sixteenth centuries, and modern-day scientists have been unable to identify the cause of the disease. The author does say that the doctors in fifteenth and sixteenthcentury England were mystified by the sweating sickness, but far from suggesting the scientists have begun to understand the disease, the author says clearly that its cause remains a mystery. Additionally, the author mentions that the disease broke out in England in the fifteenth and sixteenth centuries and has not been a problem since, but this is only the content of the first paragraph and ignores the second and third paragraphs entirely; what is more, this summary does not represent the larger point that the author is trying to make about the disease remaining a mystery for scientists. Finally, the author suggests that modern-day scientists have begun to narrow down the options (by presenting the theories about the disease), but there is nothing in the passage to indicate that fifteenth and sixteenth century doctors failed to report on the disease. In fact, in the third paragraph the author mentions doctors of the time who "wrote about the disease," and this clearly indicates that there was reporting on the disease at the time.

44. B: Answer choice B represents a theory about the sweating sickness, that it was caused by a hantavirus. This remains a theory, however, and does not represent a detail from the passage. The other answer choices, on the other hand, do represent details contained in the passage. The author notes in the first paragraph that the sweating sickness struck quickly and often killed victims within a few hours. The author says in the third paragraph that doctors in the fifteenth and sixteenth centuries did not write about seeing any bites from lice or ticks on patients. And the author notes in the first paragraph that the sweating sickness "disappeared from England in the 1570s," which is certainly the latter part of the sixteenth century.

45. D: The author makes several points in the second paragraph: (1) scientists tend to look first to hygiene and sanitation as a cause for epidemics, (2) these tend to be the greatest concern among the poor, (3) the wealthy tend to have better access to good hygiene and sanitation, and (4) the sweating sickness was more likely to strike the wealthy. Taken together, these suggest that the sweating sickness did not result from bad hygiene and sanitation among the poor. As indicated, the author says that the sweating sickness was known for striking the wealthy over the poor. In the final paragraph, the author points out that the sweating sickness is believed to have been spread by human contact. And in the first paragraph, the author states that the deaths from the sweating sickness were not as high as deaths from other epidemics in England (but that the mystery surrounding the disease made it more frightening to people).

46. B: Answer choice B is the only option to contain clearly stated information from the passage. The author says in the third paragraph that hantaviruses are carried by rodents and spread to humans when humans come in contact with the rodents or their waste. The author says nothing about hantaviruses being connected to hygiene and sanitation. The author states clearly in the third paragraph that as far as scientists know hantaviruses cannot be spread from human to human (but only when humans are around rodents or rodent waste). And the author indicates in the third paragraph that the theory of the hantavirus is the "latest theory," but that there are problems with it; these problems make it impossible to say at this time that a hantavirus was the most likely cause.

47. C: The uncertainty of the cause remains a problem for doctors and scientists: if they do not know what caused the sweating sickness, they cannot guarantee that it will not be a problem in the future, and they have no immediate way of preventing it. The author says nothing about modern medical treatments, so answer choice A cannot be correct. The author mentions that doctors in the fifteenth and sixteenth centuries did not notice the bites of lice and ticks on victims of the sweating sickness; there is nothing to suggest that they would not have the observational skills necessary to see these signs. And the author makes no mention of survivors of the disease. This does not mean that people did not survive, nor can it be argued that a low number of deaths indicates a high number of survivals. Instead, this is simply not a part of the passage.

VocabularyandGeneralKnowledgeAnswerKeyandExplanations

1. C: To *bifurcate* is to split into two parts. Within the other answer choices, there is no word with a close enough meaning: to *close* (or shut out), to *glow* (or be illuminated), and to *speak*.

2. C: An *influx* is an arrival in large amounts. For instance, the early twentieth century brought an *influx* of immigrants to the United States through Ellis Island. The word *acceptance* suggests approval, which is not contained in the meaning of *influx* (as there can also be an *influx* of something that is not acceptable). The word *complexity* is related to a degree of complication, and there is nothing in this to connect it to the meaning of *influx*. The word *theory* relates to a proposed idea. Again, there is nothing in this to suggest a clear relationship with *influx*.

3. C: To *substantiate* is to bring evidence to something and thus to *confirm* it. One who *substantiates* a claim confirms its validity. To *inhibit* is to prevent or hold back; this suggests an opposite meaning to *substantiate*. To *assume* is to believe something—with or without *substantiation*. Because *substantiate* indicates the presence of clear supporting evidence, the word *assume* (which suggests the lack of it) cannot be a synonym. To *complete* is to fulfill or accomplish a goal. There is not enough in this meaning to establish a clear relationship with *substantiate*.

4. D: The best definition for the word *typify* is *symbolize*. To *typify* is to indicate a type or *symbol*, to characterize or show an example of. To *obscure* is to make something less clear. Since the act of *typifying* indicates a goal of clarifying, the word *obscure* represents an antonym. To *mock* is to make fun of. There is not enough in the meaning of *typify* to suggest a purpose of *mockery*, so answer choice B cannot be correct. To *announce* is to share important information. There is nothing in this meaning to connect it to the meaning of *typify*.

5. C: The word *sinuous* suggests something that is winding, twisting, or *supple*. The word *ominous* has a negative connotation of impending danger, and while some *sinuous* things can also be *ominous* (such as a *sinuous mountain road that winds up to the very top*), the foundational meaning of the word *sinous* is unrelated to danger. The word *spoiled* suggests overindulgence (in a child) or a state of being rotten (in food). There is nothing in this to connect it to the meaning of *sinuous*. The word *elaborate* suggests a state of complexity. Once again, there is not enough in the meaning of the word *sinuous* to make this connection without a causal relationship.

6. B: The word *insidious* indicates someone or something that behaves in a *subtle* way, often with a negative purpose or effect in mind. The meaning of *insidious* has no relationship with the meaning of the word *loyal*, as the latter suggests dependability, while the former suggests a measure of unpredictability. Someone or something that is *insidious* might also be *intelligent*, but there is not enough in the meaning of *insidious* to assume a direct synonym. Something *unlikely* is improbable. Again, there is not enough in this to indicate a clear connection to the meaning of *insidious*.

7. D: The word *emaciated* indicates someone or something that is *wasted* from lack of nourishment. The words *vivid* and *fresh* are, to some degree, antonyms, because they indicate a state of being that is healthy and well-nourished. The word *grateful* suggests a positive response to something that is done or given, and this has no immediate relationship with the meaning of *emaciated*.

8. A: Something *irrevocable* cannot be revoked and is thus *binding*. The word *fortunate* indicates that something good has occurred or will occur. While an *irrevocable* decision might also be a *fortunate* one, it might just as easily be (and is often viewed as being) *unfortunate*. The word *unfeasible* means that something is not likely or practical. This has no immediate connection to the meaning of the word *irrevocable*. The word *indefinite* suggests a lack of certainty. This is the opposite of the implied meaning in *irrevocable*, so the words are antonyms instead of synonyms.

9. D: To *abate* is to lessen, decrease, or *reduce*. The opposite of *abate* is *enhance*, since the latter suggests an increase instead of a decrease. To *remove* is to take something away. To *abate* might require that something be taken away, but the meanings are not similar enough, giving the words a conditional relationship. To *revive* is to bring back to life or add to something. Like the word *enhance*, this has a suggestion of increase, making it a possible antonym for *abate*.

10. D: To *extirpate* is to *remove* altogether. The word *assist* suggests help, and there is nothing in here to connect it to the meaning of *extirpate*. The word *define* refers to offering a description or explaining an inherent quality. Again, there is little within this to connect it to the meaning of *extirpate*. The word *provide* indicates an addition or an increase. This makes the word *provide* an antonym for the word *extirpate*.

11. A: Someone who is *feckless* is *incompetent* or ineffective. Someone or something *significant* is of great purpose, so this represents an antonym for *feckless*. Similarly, someone or something *relevant* has immediate purpose and competency, so the word *relevant* is also an antonym. Someone or something that is *headstrong* is stubborn to the point of getting his/hers/its way. Someone *feckless* could also be *headstrong*, but there is not enough in the meanings of these words to suggest an immediate relationship.

12. C: To *constrict* is to *tighten* to an extreme. For instance, the *boa constrictor* squeezes the life out of its prey. The word *collect* indicates an amassing or assembling of items or people. To *collect* is to bring together; to *constrict* is to squeeze forcefully. This has no immediate connection with the meaning of the word *constrict*. To *appreciate* is to show gratefulness for something. Again, there is nothing in this meaning to connect it to the meaning of *constrict*. To *mingle* is to *join*. This has no clear connection to the meaning of the word *constrict*.

13. B: To *goad* is to *force* into action. To *create* is to bring into existence something new. To *bore* is to fail to generate interest for someone or something. To *please* is to make happy. None of these answer choices has any clear relationship with the meaning of the word *goad*.

14. A: The context of the sentence indicates that the school provost chose the proposal that was most *dominantly* favored among the board members. There is nothing in the context of the sentence to suggest that any proposal was deemed *old-fashioned*, so this answer choice cannot be correct. The word *indifferent* makes little sense when applied in place of *prevalent*. (To be *indifferent* is not to care, so it makes no sense for the board members to have an *indifferent favorite* or for the provost to choose a proposal for that reason.) The word *scarce* suggests lack, and since the context of the sentence indicates that the provost chose the proposal that was of interest to most, answer choice D cannot be correct.

15. C: To be *nonchalant* is to be *unconcerned* about an experience, event, or the results of something. The opposite of *nonchalant* is *excited*, so answer choice A cannot be correct. Someone who is *nonchalant* has little emotion about something. Someone who is *cowardly* has strong emotion *not* to do something, so the two words suggest a lack of activity for entirely different reasons. To be *imprudent* is to be unwise about something. A *nonchalant* person might also be *imprudent*, but there is nothing within the meanings of the two words to make an immediate connection.

16. C: To *malinger* is to falsify an illness or *pretend* that is has occurred. To *meet* is to encounter and get to know someone or something. To *prevent* is to hinder something from occurring. To *surge* is to generate a sudden increase. None of these words has any clear connection in meaning with *malinger*.

17. D: Something that is *serrated* has a *jagged* edge. An *unusual* object might also happen to be *serrated*, but a *serrated* edge is not necessarily an *unusual* feature. Someone or something *defiant* is rebellious and ignores or flaunts the rules. There is nothing in this meaning to establish a clear relationship with the meaning of the word *serrated*. Someone or something that is *sad* is in low spirits or is unhappy. The word *serrated* suggests a largely physical quality, while the word *sad* suggests a largely emotional quality. The two words have virtually no similarity in meaning.

18. B: Something *contiguous* is directly next to something else, or is *adjacent*. It is possible for the state of *adjacency* to be *unique*, but this is a largely conditional relationship, and the words have no immediate connection in meaning. Something *indirect* is out of the way or even peripheral. This means that *indirect* functions as a kind of antonym for *contiguous*, which indicates a more immediate relationship between two things. To be *pleased* is to be delighted at the results. There is little within this meaning to connect the words *pleased* and *contiguous*.

19. C: To *obfuscate* is to obscure or *conceal*. To *resemble* is to demonstrate a likeness, so this functions as an antonym for *obfuscate*. To *decide* is to make a choice. There is little in this to suggest an immediate relationship with *obfuscate*. To *surpass* is to exceed or go beyond. Again, there is little clear connection between the word *surpass* and the word *obfuscate*.

20. D: To *portend* is to *forecast* something negative. For instance, in films the ominous music often *portends* frightening events that are about to occur. To *withdraw* is to remove or take away in some form. To *deny* is to claim that something is untrue. To *uncover* is to reveal. None of these answer choices demonstrates any immediate connection to *portend*.

21. C: The context of the sentence indicates that Nina wants to speak privately to her supervisor about his comments but is concerned about *challenging* his authority before the other employees. While discussing the matter with the supervisor at the meeting might very well *disturb* him, the context of the sentence suggests that Nina's motivation stems from her desire not to embarrass her supervisor in public. The sentence clearly states that Nina is *disappointed* by the remarks, so it makes little sense for her to *encourage* her supervisor, either publicly or privately, for the comments that were made. The word *present* makes no sense in the context of the sentence and only confuses the meaning.

22. A: Something that is *immutable* has no mutability or changeability and is thus *unchangeable*. Something that is *breakable* can, by its very nature, be changed, so answer choice A represents a kind of antonym for the word *immutable*. The word *desirable* suggests a state of being wanted, and this has no clear connection to the state of being *unchangeable*. The word *flexible* indicates changeability, so this too is an antonym for *immutable*.

23. B: Something that is *protracted* has been *extended* beyond its expected limits. For instance, a *protracted* legal battle might drag out for years. Something that is *required* is necessary. Something that is *elevated* is raised up, either literally or metaphorically. Neither of these words has any immediate connection to the meaning of *protracted*. Something that is *delayed* is late or has been put on hold. In some contexts, this suggests a possible antonym for the word *protracted*.

24. D: Something that is *viable* has life within it, has options, and has a future. In other words, it is *living*, either literally or figuratively. Something that is *inanimate* has no life within it, so this is an antonym for *viable*. Something that is *reasonable* makes sense or falls within the boundaries of rational explanation. Something that is *likely* is expected to occur. Neither of these words has any direct connection to the meaning of *viable*.

25. C: To be *incessant* is to be *constant* and without ceasing (or cessation). To be *complicated* is to be difficult or convoluted. To be *uncertain* is to be without certainty and lacking definition. To be *frightening* is to be scary or alarming. None of these words has a meaning with any connection to the meaning of *incessant*.

26. C: Something that is *negligible* has little value, is insignificant, or is *minor*. The word *adequate* suggests an acceptable or approved amount; this could function as a possible antonym for *negligible*. Similarly, the word *significant* means the very opposite of the word *negligible*, so it is an antonym. The word *careless* suggests someone who *neglects* to pay attention to responsibility, but the word *neglect* and the word *negligible*, while related in origin, have entirely different meanings.

27. A: To *accost* is to *confront* or challenge someone. A person who *accosts* someone else might very well *insult* or *mock* the other person at the same time, but the verb *accost* does not have the immediate implication of a negative confrontation. In some cases, to *accost* is to issue a justifiable demand. To *evade* is to avoid, and this is the very opposite meaning of *accost*.

28. C: To *retreat* is to back off or *withdraw*. For instance, an army that *retreats* pulls its soldiers back from battle. To *provide* is to offer or give necessary or useful items. To *anger* is to cause wrath in someone else. There is no clear relationship between the meanings of either of these words and the meaning of *retreat*. To *contain* is to hold on to something or *enclose* it. The word *retreat* has the implication of getting out or getting away, so the word *contain* represents a kind of antonym for *retreat*.

29. D: A *dichotomy* is a *split* between two items or ideas. In politics, there is often a clear *dichotomy* between those on the right and those on the left. The word *formation* suggests the start of something. There is nothing in the meaning of this word to indicate a connection to the meaning of *dichotomy*. The word *decision* indicates a clear choice; while someone might make a *decision* about which side of a *dichotomy* to support, these words have a causal relationship rather than a synonymous one. The word *interruption* indicates a pause, even a *split* in time. But this stretches the possibility of a synonym for *dichotomy*. A *dichotomy* is a true split, as if with a cleaver (whether literal or metaphorical). There is the implication of a chasm between the two sides. An *interruption* is simply a pause that may or may not be filled with something else. For instance, one person who *interrupts* another often does so by jumping in and adding something of his or her own.

30. B: To be *solicitous* is to be *attentive*, often to the point of the attention being unpleasant, although there is not necessarily a purely negative quality in the word; a nurse who is *solicitous* is carefully *attentive* to his or her patients. The word *plentiful* suggests excess, and while a *solicitous* person can be described as *plentiful* in attention, the word *plentiful* is not always related directly to attention. Someone who is *ignorant* has limited knowledge and is thus not paying attention at all. This functions as a kind of antonym for *solicitous*. Someone who is *stubborn* refuses to go along with what is asked or required. There is no clear relationship between the word *stubborn* and the word *solicitous*.

31. A: A *trajectory* is a proposed *direction* that someone or something can take. A college graduate's future career can have an expected *trajectory* (where the graduate intends to go and how he or she intends to proceed in the career). A missile can have an expected *trajectory* (striking what it is supposed to strike). The word *excitement* relates to eager anticipation over some expected event. While both *excitement* and *trajectory* have an implied suggestion of anticipation, there is little else to connect the meanings of the words. The word *simplification* means a reduction down to the bare basics. There is nothing in this to suggest a clear relationship with the word *trajectory*. And while determining a *trajectory* requires a certain amount of *calculation*, the connection between these words is largely causal.

32. D: Something that is *unwarranted* is unnecessary or even *inappropriate*. Clearly, Agnes's comment is not acceptable, so the teacher calls her out for it. If the comment is *inappropriate*, it is certainly not *justifiable*, so the latter word is an antonym for *unwarranted*. Agnes's comment might be rooted in a measure of *bias*, making it *inappropriate*, but this suggests a cause-and-effect relationship instead of a synonymous one. If Agnes's remark is *unwarranted*, it is definitely not *essential*, so answer choice C cannot be a synonym.

33. A: To be *intemperate* is to lack any sense of personal restraint and thus to be *unrestrained*. For example, the Temperance Movement in the United States began in an effort to help people restrain themselves against overconsumption of alcoholic beverages (and ultimately evolved into a no-alcohol policy). Someone who is *unconcerned* is largely indifferent to what is happening. This has no clear connection with the meaning of *intemperate*. Someone who is *idle* is doing nothing and wasting time. While this meaning is not directly opposite the meaning of *intemperate*, the word *intemperate* does suggest some form of excess action—and the word *idle* suggests no action at all. To be *organized* is to be prepared, have everything planned, and even have a sense of control. This suggests a type of antonym for *intemperate*, since one who is *unrestrained* is certainly not *organized*.

34. C: Something that is *onerous* represents a great burden and is, as a result, very *demanding*. Something *trivial* is small and unimportant, making this word a kind of antonym for *onerous*. Something *motivating* encourages action; it might require *motivation* to complete an *onerous* task, but the relationship between these words is essentially causal rather than synonymous. Something that is *urgent* requires immediate attention. Again, it might be possible for something *onerous* to be *urgent* as well, but this indicates a cause-and-effect relationship instead of a direct similarity in meanings.

35. A: *Heterogeneous* indicates a measure of *difference*, things that are unique or distinct. (This is contrasted with *homogeneous*, which suggests direct similarity.) Something *heterogeneous* might also be *unusual*, but there is nothing *unusual* in the fact of *heterogeneity*. The word *clear* indicates something obvious or easy to understand. There is nothing in this meaning to suggest a similarity to the meaning of the word *heterogeneous*. The word *comparable* indicates a measure of sameness; this functions as an *antonym* for *heterogeneous*.

36. A: To be *overwrought* is to be pushed to an extreme, to be very *agitated*. To be *respected* is to bear the appreciation of peers and others. There is little in the meaning of this word to suggest a relationship with the word *overwrought*. To be *indifferent* is to lack interest or not to care about something; someone who is *overwrought* cares very much about what is happening, so the word *indifferent* represents an opposite for the word *overwrought*. One who is *overwrought* is *excessive* in emotion and concern. At the same time, it is possible to see *excess* in many other areas, so the word *excessive* describes the word *overwrought*. The two words are not, however, synonyms.

37. B: Someone who is in his or her *dotage* is in a state of *senility*. *Senility* suggests a certain weakness, so the word *strength* is a kind of antonym for the word *dotage*. The word *balance* also indicates a measure of well-being, so there is a hint of an opposite in this word as well. The word *position* indicates a role that is played; there is no immediate relationship between the word *position* and the word *dotage*.

38. D: The word *puerile* has its roots in the Latin word for *child*. As it has evolved in English usage, the word *puerile* now suggests someone who is *childish* in behavior, with a negative denotation of immaturity. The word *youthful* has a positive connotation of being young, healthy, even *childlike*—to the same thing as *childish*—so it is not a strong synonym for *puerile*. To be *sophisticated* is to have a measure of maturity; this functions as a kind of antonym for *puerile*. To be *virtuous* is to be morally upright; there is little in this meaning to connect the words *virtuous* and *puerile*.

39. C: Something that is *putative* is assumed or *accepted*, with or without solid evidence. Something or someone that is *chosen* has the mark of preference; there is little in this to connect the meaning of the word *chosen* with the meaning of the word *putative*. Something *factual* has solid support and evidence. Since *putative* indicates *acceptance*, with or without *fact*, the words are closer to being antonyms than synonyms. To be *effective* is to be useful in some form. There is no immediate relationship between this word and the word *putative*.

40. D: To *enumerate*, from the Latin "to number" or "to count," suggests a measure of clear *specification*. A patient might ask a doctor to *enumerate* the steps that he or she should take for better health. This is a request for *specific* details, not vague ideas. To *refuse* is to reject in some form. To *plead* is to beg. To *include* is to bring someone or something in. None of these words has any direct relationship in meaning to the meaning of the word *enumerate*.

41. B: Something that is *intangible* is unclear, lacking in substance, or *vague*. Something that is *sudden* is unexpected; it is possible for something to be *intangible* and *sudden*, but the relationship between the words is causal rather than synonymous. Something that is *forthright* is straightforward; this can function as a possible antonym for *intangible*. Similarly, something that is *definite* is clear; this is a strong antonym for *intangible*.

42. D: A *relapse* is a decline, a reversion of the good, or a *setback*. *Prevention* is useful to avoid a *setback*, but this relationship is more one of cause and effect (or even chronology). An *endearment* is a presentation of fondness, so there is no clear relationship between this word and the word *relapse*. A *progression* is a moving forward; this is the opposite of *relapse*, so the words are antonyms.

43. C: Something that is *definitive* is clear and precise; it can also suggest an *ultimate* quality. Something *absurd* is ridiculous. It is possible for an *absurdity* to be *definitive*, but the relationship between these words suggests cause and effect. Something that is *definitive* suggests a measure of completion, so the word *incomplete* is a kind of antonym. It is possible to *prefer* something *definitive*, but the quality of being *definitive* does not guarantee *preference*.

44. B: To *conflate* is to *merge* in some form. There is nothing about the inherent meaning of *conflation* that suggests *falsification*, so the two words are unrelated, either as antonyms or as synonyms. To *anticipate* is to expect something. Again there is nothing in this meaning to suggest a connection to the meaning of the word *conflate*. To *conflate* is to bring together; this bringing together might or might not suggest *expansion*, but *expansion* does not always come about through *conflation*.

45. D: A *congenital* condition is *innate* or in existence from birth. A *contracted* condition is one that is caught rather than inherent, so these words are antonyms. A *congenital* condition is likely to be a *lifelong* one, but the meaning of *lifelong* does not equate directly to *innateness*. For instance, someone can *contract* an illness that causes *lifelong* problems. Something *additional* is in excess. A *congenital* quality is *innate* for the one who experiences it, so it cannot be said to be *additional*.

46. A: To *gestate* is to *conceive* or begin in some form. To *provide* is to give or offer something. To *delete* is to remove something. To *remind* is to bring back to memory something that has (potentially) been forgotten. None of these words have any direct connection in meaning to the meaning of *gestate*.

47. D: Something that is *mordant* is biting in tone or *disrespectful*; to issue *mordant* criticism is to criticize in an offensive way. Something *elegant* is *sophisticated* or *graceful*—not necessarily an antonym for the word *mordant*, but it is unlikely that the qualities of *mordancy* and *elegance* would coexist. Something that is *soothing* is kind or gentle; this is a kind of antonym for the word *mordant*. Something that is *joking* is playful and not serious; to be *joking* can also be biting or *disrespectful*, but it does not necessarily have to be. The words cannot be synonyms.

48. C: To *transmute* is to *change* in some way. To *annoy* is to irritate; to *maintain* is to preserve or continue; to *charge* is to burden, allege, or establish a price on something. None of these words offers a clear connection in meaning to the word *transmute*.

49. B: To *circumscribe* is to go around and hold in, to confine, and to *enclose*. To *continue* is to keep going in some way. To *converse* is to engage in conversation. These words are unrelated in meaning to the word *circumscribe*. To *permit* is to allow; because *circumscription* suggests prevention or hindrance, the word *permit* is an antonym for the word *circumscribe*.

50. C: The word *prehensile*, with a Latin root meaning "to grasp," indicates *greed*. A *gentle* person is kind and gracious. While the words are not antonyms, it is not likely that a *gentle* person would also be *prehensile*. A *clever* person is intelligent and quick-witted. There is nothing in this meaning to suggest a connection to the meaning of *prehensile*. A *gracious* person is generous, so the words *gracious* and *prehensile* are antonyms.

GrammarAnswerKeyandExplanations

1. B: To *imply* is to give a suggestion; to *infer* is to receive that suggestion. In this sentence, Detective Melchior tries to *imply* something to his sidekick, but the sidekick cannot *infer* the meaning (i.e., the sidekick does not understand the suggestion). Answer choice B places the words in the correct order: *imply, infer*.

2. C: A sentence that is in the active tense has the subject *doing* the action instead of *receiving* it. The opposite of active tense is passive tense: the subject is receiving the action or *being acted upon*. In answer choice C, the fashion designer is *presenting* the collection—that is, he is doing the action of presenting. In answer choice A, the child is receiving the gifts from friends (*was given presents by his friends*). In answer choice B, the marathon winner is receiving the medal from the awards committee (*was rewarded...by the awards committee*). In answer choice D, the duck a l'orange is in the process of being eaten—that is, the duck is being acted upon (*was quickly devoured by the eager culinary students*).

3. C: The word *much* suggests an uncountable amount, while the word *many* suggests something countable. *Time* is uncountable, so the speaker of the sentence requires the form *much*. The speaker's *tasks* are certainly countable, so he or she requires the form *many*. Answer choice C places the words in the correct order: *much, many*.

4. D: Question 4 presents a similar situation as question 3, although now it is a choice between *less* (which is uncountable) and *fewer* (which is countable). Edwina had *less* time than she anticipated, so she went to the lane that said "Ten Items or *Fewer*." Despite the signs that read *Ten Items or Less* in grocery stores across the United States, this form is actually incorrect. If the shopper can count the number of items in his or her cart, he or she will know if there are ten items or *fewer*.

5. B: Capitalization rules require that the main words that describe the official name of a conflict be capitalized. In other words, the correct form is *World War I*, with all parts capitalized. The other answer choices, with the mix of capitalized words, cannot be correct.

6. C: Capitalization rules state that prepositions do not need to be capitalized in formal names, unless those prepositions are longer than four letters. In the case of question 6, the correct form then would be *Siege of Leningrad*, with the words *Siege* and *Leningrad* capitalized. The short preposition *of* does not need to be capitalized.

7. A: The words *earth*, *sun*, and *moon* are not capitalized unless they are listed with other planets. In this sentence, the inclusion of *Saturn*, *Neptune*, and *Jupiter* requires that *Earth* and *the Sun* be capitalized (even if the word *the* is added before *Sun*). In this case, the word *the* is not necessary before *Earth* because *Earth* is being referred to among the formal names of planets. (*The Sun* is always referred to with the article.)

8. D: Question 8 asks for the correct abbreviation for *milligrams*, which is *mg*. So the doctor prescribes *4 mg* of the medication to be taken daily. Answer choices A and B are meaningless. Answer choice C prescribes *4 meters* to the patient—clearly, not what the doctor has ordered.

9. A: The phrase *Janet and* _____ is an appositive form that expands *My two friends*. Because *My two friends* is the subject of the sentence, the pronoun in the appositive phrase should be the subjective case: *she*. The form *her* is in the objective case, as is the form *them*. The form *they* is in the subjective case, but the context of the sentence calls for *two friends*, and *Janet and they* would make for more than two.

10. C: The pronoun *Somebody* is singular, so it requires a singular verb: *has*. (*Somebody has been in my house!*) The verb *have* is plural. The verbs *will* and *might* make no sense when connected directly to *been*. In both cases, the verbs need the form *have* to follow immediately before *been*. (That is, *will have been* or *might have been*.)

11. C: The context of the sentence shows that the blank follows a preposition, making the expression the object of the preposition. Pronouns that function as the object of the preposition should be in the objective case: *us students*. (To check for sure, simply remove the word *students* since it acts as a kind of appositive and is not essential to the meaning of the sentence: *the financial burden placed on us*.) The form *we* is subjective in case. The form *those* makes no sense, as the speaker is the head of the student council and thus also a student. The form *them students* is never correct.

12. A: The rules of hyphenation require a hyphen after the first word to indicate that it should be attached to another word: *part- and full-time*, because this would otherwise be *part-time and full-time*. The hyphens are required to indicate that the combination of the two words represents a single adjective. The slashes are never used to create adjectives.

13. C: The word *take* suggests direction away from someone, and the word *bring* suggests direction toward someone. In other words, the speaker wants the person hearing him or her to *take* the tea away and to *bring* something else. Answer choice C offers the correct order of these words: *take*, *bring*.

14. A: The verb *ought* can work on its own, without a helping verb (such as *had* or *should*). In fact, *should* and *ought* are similar in meaning, so the expression *should ought* is largely redundant. The word *had* on its own makes little sense in the sentence.

15. C: Because the name *Sherlock Holmes* is singular, the possessive form requires an apostrophe and the letter *s* to follow: *Sherlock Holmes's*. The apostrophe alone is only correct for a word that is already plural. The apostrophe before the final *s* alters the name of *Sherlock Holmes* to *Sherlock Holme*. The lack of any apostrophe fails to recognize the context of the sentence, which calls for the possessive case.

16. B: The context of the sentence indicates a single novel that has a surprising solution for Linus. As a result, the singular possessive *mystery's* must be correct. The form *mysteries* is plural but has no possession. The form *mysteries'* is plural possessive, which the context of the sentence contradicts (in the singular *detective novel*). The form *mysterie's* is never correct.

17. D: The sentence has a plural subject—*Both Hugo and Camille*—so it requires a plural verb, *are*. The forms *is* and *was* are singular. The form *were* is plural, but the past tense of *were* contradicts the present tense indicated by *participate* later in the sentence. If Hugo and Camille *were* members of the local rotary club but no longer are, they would probably not still be participating in the annual auction.

18. A: The form *rise* is intransitive (requiring no object), while the form *raise* is transitive (requiring a noun/pronoun object). For example, we *rise* from bed every morning, but we *raise* a flag. The coach calls upon the team to *rise* to the challenge (no object) and *raise* the bar (the word *bar* representing an object) in this context. All other answer choices are incorrect for including the wrong words or order of the words.

19. D: The form *lie* is intransitive, and the form *lay* is transitive. The speaker says that the listener should not *lie* down (no object) but wait until he/she can *lay* new sheets (object: sheets). All other answer choices are incorrect for including the wrong words or order of the words.

20. A: The form *their* is a possessive pronoun; the form *they're* is a contraction for *they are*; the form *there* indicates direction or location. Answer choice A is correct because it correctly orders the words to identify *their car* (possessive pronoun identifying the owner of the car), identify that *they're [they are] going to Evan's house*, and noting that they will stay *there* (at Evan's house) until the car is repaired. All other answer choices are incorrect for including the wrong words or order of the words.

21. C: The form *between* should be used for two people, while the form *among* should be used for more than two people. Answer choice C is correct because it accurately fills the sentence in with *Between the two of us* and *among all ten of the board members*. All other answer choices are incorrect for including the wrong words or order of the words.

22. B: A colon should be used to introduce a list of items, only when the expression "the following" (or "as follows") appears before the list. Answer choice A does not include any punctuation between the introduction to the list and the list itself. Answer choice B uses a semicolon, thus creating a fragment in the second part of the sentence. Answer choice D uses a comma, which is not correct to introduce a list.

23. D: A semicolon may be used between items in a list when those items contain internal commas. In the case of cities and states, it is customary to use a semicolon between each city/state listing. Answer choice A fails to use any commas or semicolons, which creates confusion in separating the items in the list. Answer choice B uses only commas, which similarly creates confusion in separating each city/state listing. Answer choice C fails to use commas to separate the city from its respective state, which is incorrect.

24. D: Answer choice D correctly offsets the name *Matteo* with commas, thereby indicating direct address. Answer choice A only uses a comma before *Matteo*, and a comma is necessary after the name as well. Answer choice B fails to add a comma before *Matteo* but adds a semicolon after it. This only creates a fragment. Answer choice C uses a colon, but the context of the sentence does not require a colon. (Colons can be used to introduce defining qualities or characteristics. In this case, nothing is defined. The rest of the comment is simply completed after the speaker addresses Matteo by name.)

25. B: The form *beside* suggests adjacency, as in one person is standing *beside* another. The form *besides* suggests exclusion, as in everyone *besides* Anne was invited to the party. In the sentence, the form *besides* belongs in the first blank because only Marine and Elsa want to go to the pool. The form *beside* belongs in the second blank because Marine and Elsa plan to get some sun *beside* the pool.

26. D: The comma correctly separates the two parts of the sentence with a slight pause. Having no internal punctuation is wrong, since there needs to be some sort of separation between the two phrases. As the sentence contains a single independent clause instead of two independent clauses, the semicolon only succeeds in creating two fragments. Colons are useful for introducing defining statements, but in this case the colon makes little sense, as the second part of the sentence simply completes the initial statement. (For instance, saying the first part of the sentence without the second makes very little sense.)

27. A: The sentence is interrogative, so it requires a question mark at the end. The speaker is asking Jeannette when the guests will arrive. The statement is complete in itself, and there is no sense that the speaker trails off; as a result, the ellipsis cannot be correct. The statement is a question and not a declaration, so the period at the end cannot be correct. The speaker is not commanding Jeannette or making an exclamatory statement, so the exclamation point is incorrect.

28. C: The pronoun phrase *Either...or* is singular, so the statement *Either Eleanor or Patrick* requires a singular verb. The verb *should* makes no sense in the sentence, at least without the addition of *be*. The verbs *are* and *were* are both plural.

29. D: The context of the sentence indicates that Edgar was unable to attend the function, due to the trains. As a result, the verb *would have liked*, with its hint of the past-tense conditional, fits best. The event occurred; Edgar could not attend; he *would have liked* to attend, however. The verb *had liked* does not fit the context of Edgar's being unable to attend. The verb *would like* has a future connotation that does not work in the past tense context of the sentence (with the event having occurred). The verb *was liking* has a quality of the present tense ongoing, and this does not fit the indication of the event having passed.

30. A: The verb *were* is correct because the sentence it subjunctive in tone; subjunctive statements indicate something that could be, should be, would be, but are not. In this sentence, the context suggests that the speaker should be more diligent but is not. The verb *are* does not work in the sentence in any context. The verb *am* does not fit the conditional tone that is suggested by the use of *would* in the main clause. The verb *was* is not correct in a subjunctive sentence.

31. B: This sentence is also subjunctive, as the subjunctive tense can also indicate a demand or requirement. When that occurs, the correct usage is the *to be* version of a verb, but without the *to*. In other words, *She insisted that the children be in the house no later than four o'clock.* The verb *will* *be* almost works, but the use of the strict future form *will* does not work with the conditional tone of the sentence. (The form *would* is more correct.) The verb *are* sounds awkward in the reading of the sentence. Again, the conditional tone requires a more conditional sounding verb, and *are* is a strict present tense verb. The tone of the sentence suggests an event in the future, so the past tense verb *were* makes little sense here.

32. D: The context of the sentence calls for the phrase *to be cleaned*, indicating a future activity: *The car needs <u>to be cleaned</u> before we leave for our trip*. The form *cleaned* is an incorrect colloquial usage with a past tense context. The car is certainly not going to clean itself, so the infinitive *to clean* makes no sense in the sentence. The form *cleaning* works no better than *cleaned*, although it would fit as a gerund if it had the article *a* before it: *The car needs a cleaning*.

33. A: The word in the blank is an adverb that modifies the verb *went* and answers the question *How [did he go forward]?* As a result, the correct answer is the adverb form *cautiously*. The word *caution* is a noun, and nouns cannot modify verbs. The word *cautious* is an adjective, and adjectives can only modify nouns and pronouns. The form *cautioned* is either a past tense verb or an adjective, neither of which makes sense in the context of the sentence.

34. C: The form *well* is an adverb that is always used to indicate health. In other words, *she felt well*; she cannot feel *good* when describing health. (The form *good*, however, can be used to describe how someone feels about an action or decision, i.e., *She felt good about her decision to attend the state university*.) The forms *better* and *best* are both adjectives; additionally, neither makes sense next to the word *enough*.

35. C: While the word *important* could work in some circumstances, this sentence has a clear clue to indicate the need for a word before it: the presence of the article *a*, which cannot go before a word that begins with a vowel. (Some sentences will include the option for a(n) to indicate either possibility. As that is not the case here, the student can assume that the first word in the blank must start with a consonant.) Among the answer choices, the only one that makes sense and is grammatically correct is the adverb-adjective form *really important*, with the adverb *really* modifying the adjective *important*. The expression *more important* could work, except that the use of *more* indicates a qualifier; as the sentence does not indicate what the event is *more important than*, it fits the sentence awkwardly.

36. D: The adverb form *barely* should usually modify an adjective or another adverb. In other words, the sentence suggests that Cedric *had barely any food*—indicating that *barely* modifies the adjective *any* and indicates the limited amount of food that Cedric had. The form *barely had any* modifies the verb *had*, which is fairly awkward. After all, how does one *barely have* something? (One either *has* something, or one does not.) The expression *had any* makes no sense in the sentence, especially as the context indicates that Cedric had very little (if any) food. The expression *had barely no* is never correct because both *barely* and *no* are negatives. The combination creates the dreaded double negative.

37. B: The form *prettier* should be used to compare two entities; the form *prettiest* should be used to compare three or more entities. In the first blank, Meg is one entity, while Beth and Jo are combined into a single entity for the comparison. As a result, the form *prettier* is correct here. The second blank is a comparison of all four girls individually, so Amy can be said to be the *prettiest* of them. The correct order of the words is *prettier, prettiest*.

38. B: The word *unique* cannot be qualified. Something is either *unique*, or it is not. Something cannot be *more or less unique*, as the state of uniqueness would no longer exist. This means that the only correct form can be the word *unique* by itself. The forms *a most unique* and *a more unique* both qualify the word. The form *uniquest* is not even a word.

39. D: The form *further* should be used to describe metaphorical distance; the form *farther* should be used to describe literal distance. Therefore, *He refused to consider further*[metaphorical distance] *which route to the store would be best so he would not have to go farther* [literal distance] *than necessary*. The mention of the *store* clarifies that the unnamed *he* is making a physical journey, so the correct order of the words is *further, farther*.

40. C: As with *good* and *well*, the forms *bad* (adjective) and *badly* have distinct uses when describing health versus personal feelings. In other words, the form *bad* should describe personal feelings (just as the form *good* does), while the form *badly* should describe health. And because the form *badly* is an adverb, it can be used to describe someone's activity or performance. The first blank in the sentence describes Zenaida's personal feelings: *She felt bad* (about how the child was doing). The second blank describes the child's performance: *the child was doing so badly in the math class*. The correct order of the words should be *bad, badly*.

41. A: The word *council* describes a body of people who make decisions. The word *counsel* describes the advice that is given. As a result, Jerome submitted his issue to the *council* (or a group of people) in hopes of receiving *counsel* (or advice) from them. The correct order of the words is *council, counsel*.

42. A: The word *advise* is a verb that describes the act of providing guidance. The word *advice* is the noun that describes the actual guidance that is given. This means that the speaker of the sentence is asking that someone *advise* him/her (or provide guidance) because he/she needs some helpful *advice* (actual guidance) to make a decision about a contractor. The correct order of the words is *advise, advice*.

43. D: To *elude* is to get away from in some way. (The suspect was able to *elude* the police.) To *allude* is to make a reference of some kind. (Writers often *allude* to the work of other writers.) In the sentence, the first blank suggests that true emotions *elude* (or get away from) people. The second blank indicates that a poet was trying to *allude* to (or refer to) this in his/her work. The correct order of the words is *elude, allude*.

44. B: The correct plural form of *bus*, when it refers to the vehicle that carries people, is *buses*. The form *busses* is based on the verb *buss*, which means *to kiss*. The singular form *bus* cannot be correct because the sentence clearly indicates that Carl took more than one bus. The form *bus's* is singular possessive, and this makes no sense in the context of the sentence.

45. B: The context of the sentence suggests that the material following the colon is the actual quote from the professor. This means that it belongs in quotation marks. Additionally, poetry is punctuated according to its length. In others words, a shorter poem goes in quotation marks, while a longer poem may be italicized. The sentence does not clearly indicate the length of the poem, but there are enough clues among the incorrect answer choices to deduce the correct answer. Answer choice A places the entire statement in quotation marks but does not punctuate the title of the poem in any way. Answer choice C uses double quotation marks around the professor's statement, as well as the title of the poem. Quotes within quotes require singular quotation marks, so double quotes around the poem within the double quotes around the statement are incorrect. Answer choice D places singular quotes around the statement, with double quotes around the italicized title of the poem. Very seldom are quotation marks used around italicized expressions, unless someone is stating those expressions. Because there are already quotes around the professor's entire statement, the quotes-plus-italicization is unnecessary. (Additionally, it is incorrect in standard

American punctuation to use single quotes around a standard quotation.) This leaves only answer choice B, which places the professor's statement in double quotes and italicizes the title of the poem. As a quick note, scholars are not in complete agreement about whether Pushkin's poem is long enough to be italicized. Some place the title in quotation marks, while others italicize. Because of this, the use of either italics or quotation marks—but not both at the same time—is considered acceptable.

46. D: The correct spelling is victorious.

47. D: The correct spelling is occurrence.

48. A: The second part of the sentence contrasts with the first. "However" is the most appropriate transition to use to help create that sense of contrast.

49. A: All of the sentences except sentence A contain errors. Sentences B and C contain verb errors; sentence D is a run-on sentence.

50. B: All of the sentences except sentence B contain verb errors.

MathematicsAnswerKeyandExplanations

1. B: (500 x .75) = 375

2. A: (35 +16 =51)

3. D: (4 x 4 = 16)

4. D: (A factor is a number that divides evenly into another number.)

5. C: (75 x 34 = 2550)

6. B: (853-372= 481)

7. A

8. B: (85/100) reduces to 17/20

9. B: Divide all fractions into decimals and compare

10. B: (360 degrees ÷ 3 = 120 degrees)

11. C: ($25 + $52 + $52 + $34= $163) $163 ÷ 4 = $40.75

12. A: (437.65-325.752 = 111.898)

13. A: (43.3 x 23.03 = 997.199)

14. D: (157 lbs x .06 = 9.42 lbs) 157lbs- 9.42 lbs =147.58lbs

15. B: (650 students x .65 = 422.5) 422.5 – 340 = 82.5 ≈ 83 more students

16. C: (the hundredths place is two right of the decimal point)

17. A: (to get one multiple any fraction by its reciprocal)

18. C: (300mg + 120 mg + 900mg + 900mg + 1500mg = 4840mg, 4840mg ÷ 5 = 968 mg

19. C: (6.982 rounds to 7.0) look at the 8 it rounds the 9 to a 10 which adds a one to the ones place, the 0 holds the tenths place

20. C: (change into fraction form 625/1000 then reduce)

21. A: (set up a ratio of 6/100 = 50/x) then solve by cross multiplying

22. A: Straight multiplication

23. A: Straight division

24. C: 7 2/3

25. C: Straight addition

26. C: This is a simple addition problem involving the process of carrying. Start with the ones column and add 4+7. Write down the 1 and add the 1 to the digits in the tens column: Now add 3+7+1. Write down the 1 and add the 1 to the digits in the hundreds column. Add 6+3+1 and write down 0. Add the 1 to the digits in the thousands column. Add 4+7+1 and write down the 1. Add the 1 to the digits in the ten-thousands column. Add 1+1 and write down 2 to get the answer 21,011.

27. D: This is a simple subtraction problem. Start with the ones column and subtract 5-2, then 4-3, then 6-1, then 9-6 to get 3,513.

28. D: This is a multiplication problem with carrying. Start with the ones column. Multiply 4 by each digit in above it beginning with the ones column. Write down each product: going across it will read 3572. Now multiply 6 by each of the digits above it. Write down each product: going across it will read 5358. Ensure that the 8 is in the tens column and the other numbers fall evenly to the right. Now add the numbers like a regular addition problem to get 57,152

29. A: This is a simple division problem. Divide 97 into 292. It goes in 3 times. Write 3 above the second 2 and subtract 291 from 292. The result is 1. Bring down the 9. Since 19 cannot be divided into 97, write a zero next to the 3. Bring down the 4. Drive 97 into 194. It goes 2 times.

30. A: To change this fraction into a decimal, divide 100 into 38. 100 goes into 38 .38 times.

31. C: This is a simple addition problem. Line up the decimals so that they are all in the same place in the equation, and see that there is a 6 by itself in the hundredths column. Then add the tenths column: 8+3to get 11. Write down the 1 and carry the 1. Add the ones column: 6+1 plus the carried 1. Write down 8. Then write down the 1.

32. D: This is multiplication with decimals. Multiply the 7 by 8 to get 56. Put down the 6 and carry the 5. Multiply 7 by 2 to get 14. Add the 5. Write 19 to left of 6. Multiply the 1 by the 8 to get 8. Multiply 1 by 2 to get 2. Add the two lines together, making sure that the 8 in the bottom figure is even with the 9. Get 476. Count 4 decimal points over (2 from the top multiplier and 2 from the second multiplier) and add a 0 before adding the decimal.

3 HESI Admission Assessment Practice Tests

33. C: Count from the 3: tenths, hundredths, thousandths.

34. A: Write 512 then add the decimal in the thousandths place, the third place from the right.

35. A: To add fractions, ensure that the denominator (the number on the bottom) is the same. Since it is not, change them both to 56ths. 1/8 equals 7/56. 3/7 equals 24/56. Now add the whole numbers: 3+6 = 9 and the fractions 31/56.

36. C: To subtract fractions, ensure that the denominator (the number on the bottom) is the same. Since it is not, change them both to 14ths. 1/7 = 2/14; 1/2 = 7/14. The equation now looks like this: $4\frac{2}{14} - 2\frac{7}{14}$. Change the 4 to 3 and add 14 to the numerator (the top number) so that the fractions can be subtracted. The equation now looks like this: $3\frac{16}{14} - 2\frac{7}{14}$. Subtract: $1\frac{9}{14}$

37. A: To multiply mixed numbers, first create improper fractions. Multiply the whole number by the denominator, then add the numerator. $1\frac{1}{4}$ becomes $\frac{5}{4}$; $3\frac{2}{5}$ becomes $\frac{17}{5}$; $1\frac{2}{3}$ becomes $\frac{5}{3}$.

The problem will look like this: $\frac{5}{4} \times \frac{17}{5} \times \frac{5}{3} = \frac{425}{60} = 7\frac{5}{60} = 7\frac{1}{12}$.

38. A: To divide fractions, change the second fraction to its reciprocal (its reverse) and multiply: $\frac{3}{5} \times \frac{2}{1}$

39. A: To solve, test each answer. Notice the in (A), the numerator has been multiplied by 3 to get 12. The denominator has been multiplied by 3 to get 21. In (B) the numerator has been multiplied by 4 and the denominator has been multiplied by 5. In (C), the numerator has been multiplied by 3 and the denominator has been multiplied by 4. In (D), the numerator has been multiplied by 4 and the denominator has been multiplied by a number less than 4.

40. D: The denominator has been multiplied by 3 to get 21. Think of what number multiplied by 3 totals 18.

41. C: Divide the numerator and denominator by 14.

42. A: Divide 68 by 7. The answer is 9 with a remainder of 5.

43. A: Write .36, and then move the decimal two places. Add the percent sign.

44. A: Divide 3 by 60 to get .05 or 5%

45. D: Divide 1 by 25 to get .04 or 4%.

46. A: Divide 40 by 8 to get 5. Multiply 5 by 3 to get 15.

47. D: To solve, first get both fractions on the same side of the equation to isolate the percentage sign. When $\frac{5}{6}$ is moved to the opposite side of the equation, it must be divided by the fraction there: $\frac{1}{3} \div \frac{5}{6}$ To divide one fraction into another, multiply by the reciprocal of the denominator: $\frac{1}{3} \times \frac{6}{5} = \frac{6}{15} = \frac{2}{5} = 40\%$.

48. D: To solve, divide 15 into 3.

3 HESI Admission Assessment Practice Tests

49. C: To change a fraction to a percent, multiply it by $100 : \frac{3}{12} \times \frac{100}{1}$

50. D: To solve, first write the fraction as $\frac{8}{100}$.

Reduce by dividing numerator and denominator both by 4.

BiologyAnswerKeyandExplanations

1. A: Sodium and potassium are the two key ingredients needed to transmit a message down the nerve cell. The ions move in and out of the cell to generate an action potential to convey the impulse. Once the impulse reaches the end of the neuron, calcium channels open to allow calcium to rush into the synaptic space. Actin and myosin are the two proteins that cause contraction of muscle fibers.

2. B: The answer is translocation. Nondisjunction is a genetic mutation where the chromosomes fail to separate after replication. This results in two cells with an abnormal number of chromosomes (one with too many, one with too few). Deletion is when a section of the chromosome is erased. Crossing over occurs when the two chromosomes are joined by the centromere and two of the legs cross over and switch places on the two chromosomes.

3. A: Our skin and mucus membranes are the first line of defense against potentially invading bacteria. Their purpose is to keep the bacteria from getting into the body in the first place. Any break or tear in the skin or mucus membranes can allow harmful bacteria or viruses to attack the body. Once inside, macrophages, T-cells, and lymphocytes will be summoned to attack infected body cells and the invading pathogens.

4. C: Capping the end of a mRNA strand protects the strand from degradation and "wear and tear." Such damage to a strand of mRNA could be catastrophic, as it directs the synthesis of proteins that are vital for life.

5. A: A clue here is that chlorophyll is involved, meaning this is a photosynthesis reaction. The light-dependent reaction involves a hydrolysis reaction to provide electrons to chlorophyll, and the release of oxygen molecules. During the light-independent reaction, the energy produced from the dependent reaction is stored in the form of chemical bonds in glucose molecules.

6. D: Photosynthesis is the process that plant cells use to obtain energy from the sun. Diffusion and active transport are both methods of ionic movement, but transpiration occurs when water moves up a plant's conduction tubes against the force of gravity.

7. C: Ethylene is the plant hormone that causes ripening of fruit. Auxins and cytokinins both promote cell growth. Auxins specifically encourage stem elongation and can also inhibit growth of lateral branches. Abscisic acid inhibits cell growth and seed germination.

8. D: Thigmotropism is the growth of plant structures in response to physical contact, similar to how vines will change their direction of growth to stay in contact with a wall or other item. Growth towards light is called phototropism, and gravitropism is growth of leaves and stems opposite to the force of gravity.

9. A: The stigma is a long tube that extends from the center of a flower whose function it is to gather pollen and transport it down the carpel toward the ovum. The bright colored petals of a flower help attract pollinators like birds, bees, and butterflies. Pollen is made in the stamen and anther, which protrude from the flower to make it easier for the pollinators to gather pollen as they fly from flower to flower. The ovary of the flower provides nourishment for the developing seeds.

10. B: Think the pneumonic "King Philip Came Over From Germany Swimming." This stands for kingdom, phyllus, class, order, family, genus, species. It relates the classification system for every species of plant and animal in the world. The further down the line that two species are similar, the more closely related they are. Genus is the most specific taxonomic category listed in the given answer choices, and so organisms with the same genus are most closely related.

11. B: A pioneer species is the first species to colonize a new area. Primary producers are organisms that produce their own food, usually from sunlight. Primary producers tend to be plants. Primary consumers are herbivores and eat primary producers. Secondary consumers eat primary consumers, and tertiary consumers eat secondary consumers.

12. C: Microtubules, microfilaments and intermediate filaments are all types of fibrous proteins that are found in the cytoskeleton and provide structural support. They also assist in the transport of materials and aid in cell motility. Glycoproteins are not found in the cytoskeleton.

13. D: Coniferous forests are populated by cone-bearing trees, or conifers. Tundras are very cold and harsh environments located mainly in the arctic. These biomes are characterized by very low temperatures and harsh winds. Tropical forests have a very dense population of different tree and plant species, with varying amounts of precipitation, and tend to exist around the equator. Temperate deciduous forests are found in moderate climates where there are warm summers and cold winters. During the winters, the trees will lose their leaves.

14. B: Biotic factors are living things, like plants and animals. Populations, communities, and individuals are also examples of biotic factors. The most basic abiotic factors are temperature, water, sunlight, and wind.

15. D: Detritivores eat only dead and decaying matter Herbivores eat plants, carnivores eat meat, and omnivores eat both plants and animals.

16. A: This type of growth produces an S curve, similar to "∫". Look at the shape and you can see how it starts out with a slow rise and then increases dramatically. After a rapid period of growth, the curve levels off at the top of the S shape.

17. C: When one member of a symbiotic relationship benefits and the other is harmed, it is termed parasitism. Mutualism occurs when both members benefit from the symbiotic relationship. Predation is when one member actively feeds on the other, causing death of the hunted species. During commensalism, one member of the relationship benefits and the other neither benefits nor is harmed.

18. A: The genotype for the two parents is Bb. Crossing Bb with Bb will give 75% brown mice and 25% white mice. Twenty-five percent of 24 is six white mice.

19. C: The genotype for each of the parents is RrWw. Set up a Punnett Square for the cross RrWw X RrWw. There are 16 possible outcomes: nine red eyes with wings: three red eyes without wings: three white eyes with wings: one white eye without wings.

20. B: Sex linked traits are carried on the X chromosome, which means that men are significantly more affected than women. Affected men can inherit the trait from either parent, depending on who carries the gene. Such disorders can occur in females—if both parents carry the trait and pass it on to their daughter—but it is very rare.

21. D: Prokaryotic cells are single-celled organisms that don't have a formal nucleus. Pili and flagella are external structures that help the cell move around. Pili are a small arm-like protrusion that can stick to other surfaces; flagella are long whip-like structures that move in a rapid fashion to propel the cell forward. A capsule is a sticky coating that some cells secrete to help the cell stick to a surface and can even provide some degree of protection. Most cells have a rigid outer cell wall (external to the plasma membrane) that provides a great deal of protection for the cell.

22. A: Enzymes are proteins that facilitate reactions, making it easier or even possible for the reaction to occur. There are several factors that can affect how well the enzyme functions: temperature, pH of the environment, and concentration of the enzyme or substrate. In addition, the presence of other proteins, called competitive or noncompetitive inhibitors will have a direct impact on enzymatic function.

23. B: The process of transcription is the conversion of DNA into mRNA, which is a complementary form of the original DNA strand. That means that mRNA is formed with the opposite bases. For example, a DNA strand of CGATGA would form an mRNA strand of GCUACU. In RNA, the base uracil is used instead of thymine. Transcription allows the ribosome to read the information coded in DNA to form proteins.

24. C: Translation is the process of reading a strand of mRNA and assembling the amino acid chain according to the information encoded on that strand. This process takes place in the ribosome.

25. D: Stabilizing selection occurs when the intermediate form of a trait, rather than the extreme form, is being selected for. Directional evolution tends to favor one of the extreme forms of the trait so that eventually, the trait typically becomes more apparent and more extreme as time goes on. Both convergent and divergent evolution refers to patterns of evolution among groups of species. Divergent evolution occurs when groups of species with a common ancestral trait evolve into different adaptations over time. Convergent evolution refers to when species that aren't related to each other develop similar traits independently of each other.

ChemistryAnswerKeyandExplanations

1. C: Use the equation, $[H^+] = 10^{-pH}$, to find that the concentration of hydrogen ions is 10^{-7}. The pH of a neutral solution is 7.

2. B: Adding an acid to a base will always yield water and a salt. It is difficult to determine the pH of the resulting solution because it depends on how acidic and basic the two initial solutions are.

3. D: Alcohols are classified by the presence of a hydroxyl group (oxygen bound to a hydrogen atom). Compounds with nitrogen bonded to other carbon atoms are called amines and are further classified according to how many carbons are attached to the nitrogen. A carbon atom with a double bond to an oxygen atom and a single bond to a hydroxyl group is the functional group of carboxylic acids. Benzene rings are an example of an aromatic hydrocarbon.

4. B: Amines are classified by the number of carbon atoms the nitrogen is bonded to. In a primary amine, nitrogen is bound to one carbon (designated by R functional group). In secondary and tertiary amines, the nitrogen is bound to two and three carbons respectively. Choice A is an example of a ketone.

5. D: Hydrocarbons are a class of molecules that contain only hydrogen and carbon. They tend to be volatile and reactive, with low boiling and melting points. London dispersion forces are present in every molecule, and hydrocarbons are no exception. Hydrocarbons tend to be gases at room temperature, not solids.

6. A: Ketones and aldehydes are very similar structurally. They each have a double bond between carbon and oxygen. In ketones, there are two functional bonds to the central carbon, while in aldehydes there is only one functional group and a hydrogen atom bound to the central carbon. They both have some properties of nonpolar and polar compounds.

7. C: A substitution reaction occurs in hydrocarbons when one of the hydrogen atoms is replaced with a different atom. When a radical, or highly reactive compound or atom, reacts with and bonds to an unpaired electron in any open shell, it is called a radical reaction. Hydrolysis and condensation are almost exactly opposite. Hydrolysis refers to when a water molecule is added to a compound to break it apart. Condensation occurs when water is released after two groups bond together.

8. D: These are called resonance structures. The double bond can occupy any of these positions and rather than alternate between these three different structures, the molecule is actually a hybrid of all three at once. It is said that there are three 1 ⅓ bonds between the oxygen and nitrogen molecules.

9. B: Positron emission and electron capture are both examples of radioactive decay processes, which release radioactive particles. Using these theories of radioactive decay can lead to extreme energy production. Nuclear fission is the process when a neutron bombards and splits open a nucleus. Fusion occurs when hydrogen atoms combine to form helium and electrons, releasing a tremendous amount of energy, far more than fission reactions.

10. D: The noble gases, group 18 on the periodic table, have a full valence shell of 8 electrons. This is significant because it means that the gases are completely inert and unable to form compounds with other elements.

11. A: This is Avogadro's number, and needs to be memorized. One mole is 6.022×10^{23} units of anything. It is a commonly used constant.

12. B: To convert from Fahrenheit to Celsius, simply subtract 32 from the Fahrenheit temperature and divide the result by 1.8. Next, to convert from Celsius to Kelvin, add 273 to the Celsius temperature. 99.1° F $= 37^\circ$ C $= 310$ Kelvin.

13. A: To solve this problem, you would need to use Boyle's law, which states that $P_1V_1 = P_2V_2$. Filling in the appropriate variables gives you $(35)(x) = (2.5)(100)$. Solve for x to find that the initial pressure was 0.875 atm.

14. C: According to the ideal gas law, $PV = nRT$, the pressure of the gas will decrease as the volume increases. This is because there will be the same amount of gas but in a larger space. According to Charles' Law, temperature and volume are directly related. This means that as the volume of the gas increases, the temperature of the gas will increase as well. Increasing the volume of the gas will have no effect on the number of moles or volatility.

15. D: A covalent bond forms between two atoms when the electron pair forming the bond are shared between the two atoms. When both shared electrons come from the same atom, it is called a coordinate covalent bond. An ionic bond forms when one electron is actually transferred from one atom to the other during the process.

16. B: During a combustion reaction, light and heat are released as water and carbon dioxide are formed. It is a rapid and often violent reaction that usually occurs in the presence of oxygen.

17. C: Colligative properties are properties that depend on the amount of solute in a solution. The elevation of a solution's boiling point, depression of its freezing point, and vapor pressure are all examples of a colligative property. If solute is added to the solution, the degree of depression or elevation changes in relation to the amount of solute added.

18. D: To balance the carbon atoms in the above equation, you must place a 6 in front of the molecule of CO_2. A 6 must also be placed in front of the molecule of water to balance the hydrogen atoms. Finally, there are 18 atoms of oxygen on the right side of the equation. On the left, there are 6 atoms in the glucose molecule, so by placing a 6 in front of the oxygen molecule, the equation will be balanced.

19. B: There are three laws of thermodynamics. The first is that energy is finite and is neither created nor destroyed. The second law is that entropy, or disorder, is always increasing in the universe. The third, and final, law of thermodynamics is that there is no disorder or entropy when a perfect crystal is at absolute zero temperature. Choice D is not one of the laws of thermodynamics.

20. D: When two atoms are bonded together, they share an electron pair, or two electrons. If a double bond is formed, they share two pairs of electrons, or four electrons. Three electrons pairs or six electrons are shared in a triple bond.

21. A: When it comes to their reaction to water, molecules are either hydrophobic or hydrophilic. Hydrophobic molecules are 'afraid' (think: phobic) of water, and tend to be nonpolar and cluster together to minimize their contact with water. Hydrophilic, or water-loving, molecules are usually polar because of their ability to react with other charged molecules.

22. C: A monosaccharide is a single sugar molecule, with the basic formula of $(CH_2O)_N$ Glucose, fructose, and mannose are all examples of monosaccharides. Sucrose is a disaccharide—two sugar molecules linked together.

23. B: An exergonic reaction is one that releases energy or heat, such as combustion. These reactions tend to occur spontaneously. An endergonic reaction is one that absorbs energy and thus cannot occur unless energy is available to feed the reaction A hydrolysis reaction refers to one where a molecule of water is added across a molecule to break the molecular bonds.

24. C: There are several different ways to classify acids and bases. According to the Arrhenius definition, acids give off hydrogen ions (H^+) in a solution and bases give off hydroxide ions (OH^-) in a solution. According to the Brønsted-Lowery definition, acids also donate protons (H^+) but bases accept the protons. The Lewis definition is another classification of acids/bases, where acids have the ability to accept a pair of electrons, while the base is able to donate a pair of electrons.

25. A: London dispersion forces are weak forces that exist between all molecules and, in fact, are the only forces that are present in some compounds, such as nonpolar molecules. Dipole-dipole forces are present in dipolar compounds, which govern the behavior of these substances. There are no such forces as hydrogen forces, though hydrogen bonding occurs between hydrogen atoms and either nitrogen, oxygen, or fluorine, which form very polar compounds. Chemical bonds are the forces that bond atoms to each other and are not an example of an intermolecular force.

Anatomy and PhysiologyAnswerKeyandExplanations

1. B: The reticular activating system (RAS) is primarily responsible for the arousal and maintenance of consciousness. The midbrain is a part of the brainstem, which has a crucial role in the regulation of autonomic functions like breathing and heart rate. The diencephalon consists of the hypothalamus and thalamus in the middle part of the brain between the cerebrum and midbrain. It plays a huge role in regulating and coordinating sensory information and hormonal secretion from the hypothalamus. The limbic system tends to the major instinctual drives like eating, sex, thirst, and aggression.

2. A: The triceps reflex forces the triceps to contract, which in turn extends the arm. Eliciting the deep tendon reflexes is an important indication of neural functioning. Without them, it can be a clue to serious spinal cord or other neurological injury. The physician should be notified immediately if a patient loses deep tendon reflexes.

3. C: The acoustic nerve, or CN VIII, is responsible for hearing and balance. To test this nerve, the practitioner could test the patient's hearing in each ear and use a tuning fork to determine the patient's ability to hear and feel the vibrations.

4. A: The parathyroid glands are four small glands that sit on top of the thyroid gland and regulate calcium levels by secreting parathyroid hormone. The hormone regulates the amount of calcium and magnesium that is excreted by the kidneys into the urine.

5. D: The empty egg follicle (once the egg was ovulated) is now called the corpus luteum and secretes large amounts of progesterone. Progesterone is the primary hormone responsible for maintaining a pregnancy. Follicle stimulating hormone and luteinizing hormone have already stopped production, and estrogen decreased right before ovulation.

6. B: Insulin and glucagon are the two main options here. Insulin is produced during periods of high blood sugar and promotes glucose absorption into the cells and the storage of glucose as glycogen and lipids in the liver. Glucagon has the opposite effect; when blood sugar is low, glucagon production promotes the breakdown of glycogen into glucose.

7. D: The myocardium is the layer of the heart that contains the muscle fibers responsible for contraction (Hint: myo- is the prefix for muscle). The endocardium and epicardium are the inner and outer layers of the heart wall, respectively. The pericardium is the sac in which the heart sits inside the chest cavity.

8. C: The SA node in the right atrium generates the impulse that travels through the heart tissue and to the AV node. The AV node sits in the wall of the right atrium and coordinates atrial and ventricular contraction of the heart. The impulse then travels down to the bundle of His, the two main (left and right) branches of conduction fibers and to the Perkinje fibers which spread the impulse throughout the rest of the heart.

9. A: This is a tricky question; most of the time, veins carry deoxygenated blood and arteries carry oxygenated blood. However, in this case, the pulmonary veins carry oxygenated blood from the lungs to the heart and the pulmonary arteries carry deoxygenated blood from the heart to the lungs.

10. C: Eosinophils are most commonly recruited to deal with allergenic antigens. Monocytes, neutrophils, and basophils also deal with antigens during the immune response, but eosinophils are found to be elevated during an allergic response.

11. B: Vitamin K is stored by the liver and is essential for the synthesis and conversion of several clotting factors, including Factor II, Factor VII, Factor IX, and Factor X. Without adequate amounts of this vitamin, the clotting factors will not be able to function properly.

12. C: Afferent vessels carry fluid toward a structure; efferent vessels carry fluid away from the structure. So afferent lymph vessels carry lymph towards the node, and efferent vessels carry lymph away from the node.

13. D: Cricoid cartilage refers to the thick rings of cartilage that surround the trachea, sitting right above the voice box. The purpose of these thick rings is to serve as additional support and protection for the delicate airway.

14. A: The mediastinum is found in the middle of the thorax, right between the lungs. It contains many structures, including the heart, the upper part of the aorta, pulmonary blood vessels, the superior and inferior vena cava, the thymus, the trachea, the esophagus, and large nerves, such as the phrenic, vagus, and cardiac. The xiphoid process lies below the mediastinum.

15. B: The duodenum is the first segment of the small intestine, connecting to the stomach on one end and to the ileum on the other. The ileum sits between the duodenum and the last section of small intestine, the jejunum, which then connects to the large intestine.

16. D: There are several hormones secreted in the GI system that play a role in digestion. Gastrin encourages the secretion of other gastric enzymes and the motility of the stomach, while gastric inhibitory peptides work to inhibit gastric enzymes and motility. Secretin and cholecystokinin both stimulate the release of pancreatic enzymes and peptides that are instrumental in digestion.

17. C: Food enters the digestive system through the mouth and proceeds down to the stomach after mastication by the teeth. Once in the stomach, enzymes are secreted that begin to digest the specific substances in the food (proteins, carbohydrates, etc). Next, the food passes through to the small intestine where the nutrients are absorbed and then into the large intestine where extra water is absorbed.

18. A: The bladder capacity of an average adult is approximately 500 to 600 ml. Excess urine in the bladder would eventually cause bladder distention and the back-up of urine into the rest of the urinary system.

19. C: Anti-diuretic hormone regulates the amount of urine output from the body. When ADH is produced in large amounts, the kidneys absorb extra water, concentrating the urine. When ADH secretion slows down, the kidneys release extra water and dilute the urine.

20. B: Interstitial fluid is found in the tissues around the cells; intracellular fluid is found within the cells. Fluid in the ventricles of the brain and down into the spinal cord is called cerebrospinal fluid. Cerebrospinal fluid bathes these sensitive tissues in a fluid that helps to protect them. Blood and lymph are the fluids that carry nutrients, oxygen, waste, and lymph material throughout the body.

21. D: There is a very narrow range of normal pH values in the human body, 7.35 to 7.45. Values lower than 7.35 indicate acidosis, and pHs higher than 7.45 indicate alkalosis. The human body can't function properly if the pH is outside of the normal range.

22. A: Patients with low respiratory rate or who are retaining CO_2 are at a high risk for developing respiratory acidosis. The buildup of CO_2 will lead to an elevated $PaCO_2$. Extra CO_2 in the blood will combine with water to form carbonic acid H_2CO_3, which will disassociate to form H^+ and HCO_3-. The excess hydrogen will drop the pH. If the H_2CO_3 is also abnormal and the pH is on the low side of normal, the metabolic system is likely compensating for the respiratory abnormality. This is called "compensated respiratory acidosis."

23. B: Leydig's cells, found in the testes, secrete testosterone, which is responsible for the majority of male sexual development. Sertoli cells are also in the testes but aid in supporting developing sperm cells. Skene's glands are found in the female and are not involved in testosterone production. Cowper's glands are accessory organs that secrete fluid contributing to the seminal fluid.

24. D: Every month during a normal menstrual cycle, a single egg is released from the ovary and moves down the fallopian tubes toward the uterus. If sperm cells are in the reproductive tract, they will encounter and fertilize the egg in the fallopian tubes. The fertilized egg will subsequently travel the rest of the way into the uterus and implant in the uterine lining.

25. D: Langerhans cells and melanocytes both have protective functions, though melanocytes protect the skin against UVA and UVB radiation. Langerhans cells are found in the epidermis and assist lymphocytes in processing foreign antigens. Eccrine glands secrete sweat, which aids in temperature regulation and excretion of water and electrolytes. Reticular fibers make up part of the structure of the extracellular material.